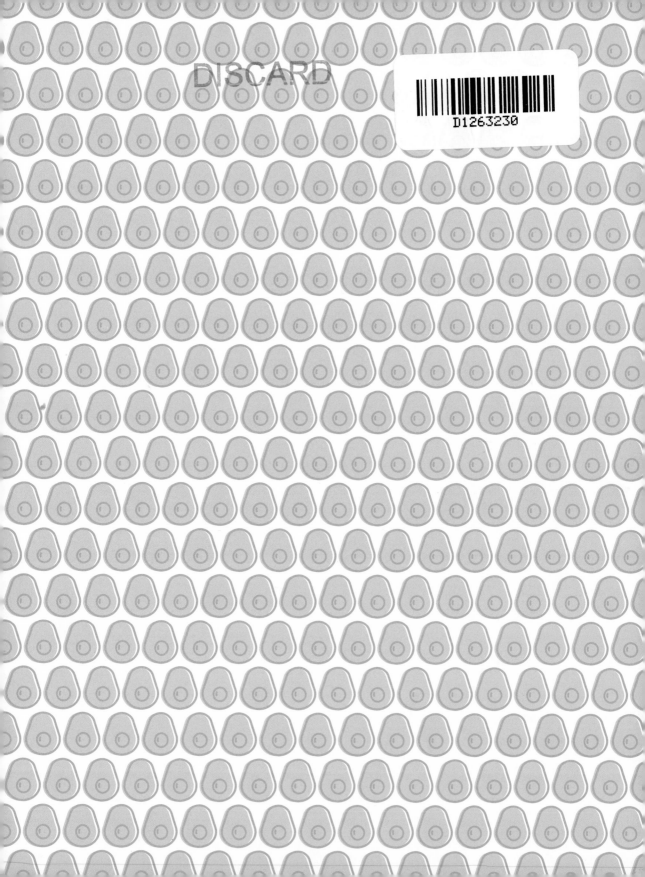

THE
WHOLESOME *yum*
EASY
KETO
COOKBOOK

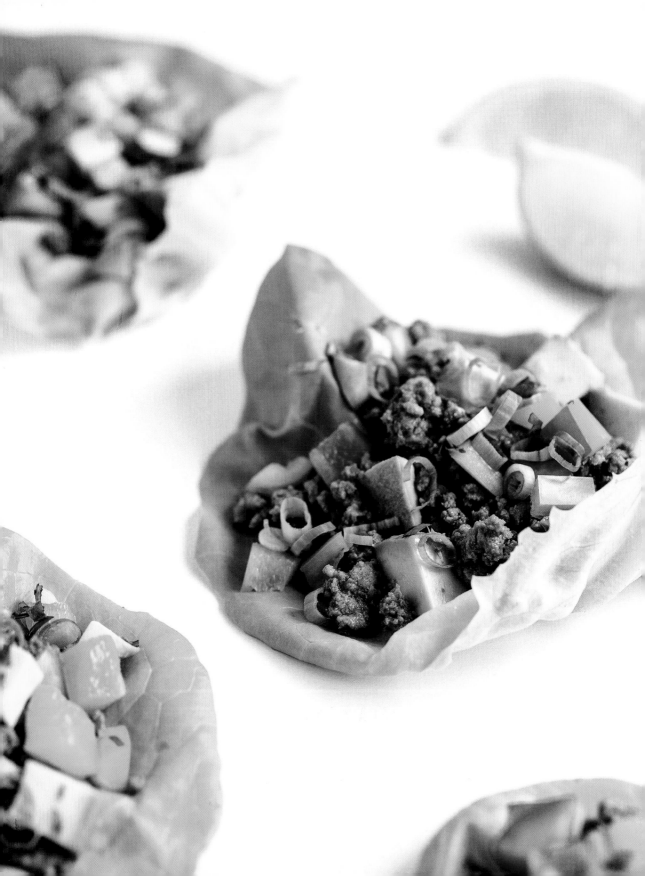

100 SIMPLE LOW CARB RECIPES. 10 INGREDIENTS OR LESS.

THE WHOLESOME *yum*
EASY
KETO
COOKBOOK

MAYA KRAMPF

HARMONY
BOOKS

NEW YORK

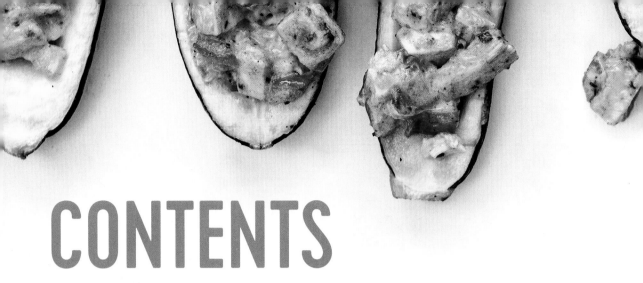

CONTENTS

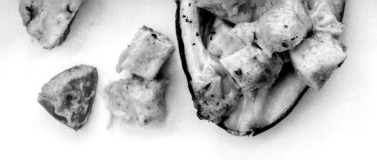
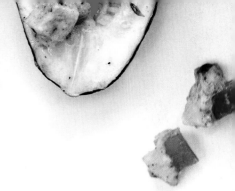

GETTING STARTED

INTRODUCTION

There's a reason that the ketogenic diet has become so wildly popular. It truly works. And, weight loss is just the beginning. Studies have shown that it stabilizes mood, raises energy levels, controls blood sugar, lowers blood pressure, improves cholesterol, and more.

I have personally seen the benefits in my own life. I spent years feeding bad habits in my teens and early twenties. This time in my life was marked with packaged foods, loads of sugar, low energy, anxiety, and even depression. Like many people, I started a low carb diet to lose weight.

Surprisingly, while the weight loss was nice, the biggest impact was the benefit to my overall health.

The low carb, keto lifestyle has completely changed my mental and physical well-being. I feel more motivated and energetic than I ever have in my life. My mood is stable. My anxiety and depression are gone. Two kids later, I'm at a healthy weight with low blood pressure and cholesterol, despite a strong family history of the contrary.

Unfortunately, many people are intimidated by keto. They don't have a lot of time to cook, they have a whole family to feed, or they worry that they'll miss their favorite meals.

I created my site, WholesomeYum.com, to show people that low carb and keto eating doesn't have to be difficult, complicated, or boring. It all started as a way to record my recipe experiments. Never in my wildest dreams did I imagine that it would help millions of people.

Every day, readers tell me how the keto lifestyle has changed their lives. My only wish is to help more people see how easy and beneficial it can be.

This book is an extension of that undertaking. It's packed with delicious and easy keto recipes, including everything you need to make them foolproof—from step-by-step instructions that even the most novice cooks can follow to great tips and variations that will help you nail each recipe and even make it your own.

Like the Wholesome Yum website, **each recipe in *The Wholesome Yum Easy Keto Cookbook* requires 10 ingredients or less**. By convention, salt and pepper are not included, and we only count each ingredient once, even if it's used twice in making a dish. And of course, each recipe includes essential macros information.

You'll also learn the basics of how to get started if you are new to a low carb or keto lifestyle. And if you aren't, you'll still find something new in these easy keto recipes!

HOW THE KETO DIET WORKS

Most followers of the keto diet prefer to call it a lifestyle—and that's because it's life-changing for so many. Benefits include weight loss, stable mood and energy levels, blood sugar control, reduced cravings and appetite, lower blood pressure, higher good cholesterol levels, glowing skin, improved digestion, and possibly increased lifespan.

But just as important, people follow this lifestyle because it's incredibly versatile and flexible.

Keto does not have to be complicated, and believe it or not, you don't have to give up your favorite foods! But you do have to shift your mindset.

If you are new to keto, it's time to throw out everything you thought you knew about how to eat. We've had it drummed into us since the low-fat diet movement began in the 1950s that fat is the enemy. But we now know that fat is not the enemy. Fat does not make you fat. Sugar does. Here's why . . .

WHAT IS THE KETO DIET?

The ketogenic diet is a high-fat, moderate-protein, low carb diet. The main difference between a keto diet and a low carb diet is that the goal of a keto diet is to get into a metabolic state called ketosis. We achieve this with the right ratio of macronutrients—fat, protein, and carbohydrates. Ketosis is the metabolic state in which we burn fat instead of sugar for fuel. To understand this, we have to understand how carbs and fat are metabolized.

HOW METABOLISM WORKS ON A HIGH-CARB DIET

When we eat carbohydrates, the body breaks them down into glucose (sugar), the primary fuel source on a standard American diet. This leads to a blood sugar spike, which triggers the pancreas to release insulin. Insulin lowers our blood sugar and signals the body to hold onto fat stores. The sugar travels from the blood into cells, giving us a short burst of energy. Some of this sugar is stored in the liver as glycogen, and the rest is converted to fat for storage. With all the sugar removed, we get a blood sugar crash, which triggers cravings, hunger, and low energy.

Even if we eat fewer calories than we need, fat loss is slow and difficult. The body in this metabolic state is not adapted to burning fat for fuel, and the frequent insulin release makes us resistant to burning body fat. Further, because the body in this state is used to burning glucose for fuel, a calorie deficit causes us to break down muscle along with fat when we do lose weight, because protein can be converted to glucose.

HOW METABOLISM WORKS ON A KETO DIET

When we restrict carbohydrates significantly, the body switches to an alternate fuel source: fat. This is called the metabolic state of ketosis. Some of this fat comes from our food, and the rest comes from fat storage. Fat travels to the liver, which breaks it down into ketones. These are units of energy that the body uses for fuel instead of glucose. They also have numerous mental and physical therapeutic effects, and tend to suppress appetite, making it easier to lose weight.

Since there is very little glucose in the system when the body is in a state of ketosis, we avoid insulin spikes. This means no signal to hold onto body fat, diminished cravings, and stabilization of energy levels and mood. (There is typically a small amount of glucose that comes from gluconeogenesis, the process of converting protein to glucose, and from the limited amounts of carbs we do eat. However, it is not the primary fuel source.) Over time, the body becomes adapted to converting fat into ketones and burning them for fuel. This makes it easy to tap into the body's fat stores and achieve real weight loss—losing fat, not muscle.

If the idea of ketosis is new to you, you may wonder if it's "normal" for the body to be in such a metabolic state. It is. It's actually quite natural. If you think about how our ancestors ate for thousands of years, their primary fuel sources were meats, vegetables, and healthy fats. Modern grains did not exist, and high-sugar fruits were sparse. Ketosis was a natural metabolic state for early humans a lot of the time.

While the keto diet is not the same as a paleo diet, there is a lot of overlap. Both diets focus on whole foods, with a lot of emphasis on healthy fats, meat, poultry, eggs, and vegetables, while eliminating grains, legumes, and processed sugars. However, the paleo diet allows high-carbohydrate natural foods such as sweet potatoes, bananas, tropical fruits, and maple syrup, while the keto diet does not. These foods are not suitable for the keto lifestyle because they spike blood sugar. On the other hand, high-fat dairy products, such as cheese and cream, are not appropriate for paleo but are keto-friendly.

One common misconception about keto is that "anything goes" as long as you stay in ketosis. This just isn't true. You may see some processed products claiming to be keto-friendly, but the healthy way to follow the keto lifestyle is a whole-foods-based approach. Keto breads and desserts are fine in moderation, but the fundamentals of the keto diet are healthy fats, unprocessed meats, eggs, and what is most often overlooked—low carb vegetables.

GETTING STARTED ON THE KETO LIFESTYLE

Now that you understand how it works, here are the basic principles for following a ketogenic diet:

1. LIMIT CARBOHYDRATES

This is the most important! The only way to get into ketosis is to restrict carbohydrates. Don't fall for the hype of ketone supplements or other gimmicks. You reach ketosis by setting a limit on carbs and not going over it, so that the body turns to fat for an alternate fuel source.

One important distinction is total carbs versus net carbs. Total carbs include fiber and sugar alcohols. Net carbs = total carbs minus fiber and sugar alcohols. Sugar alcohols are a type of natural sugar-free sweetener commonly used in a keto lifestyle. The reason we subtract these is they do not affect blood glucose levels. (Technically some sugar alcohols do have an effect, so stick to ones that do not—mainly erythritol and xylitol.) Fiber is necessary and important, and is safe to exclude from carb counts. I recommend counting net carbs when factoring in your carbohydrate limit.

MACRO TIP • **Carbohydrates are 5 to 10 percent of total calorie intake on a keto diet.** To get into and stay in ketosis, keep net carbs around 20 to 30 grams per day.

2. MEET, BUT DON'T EXCEED, YOUR PROTEIN GOAL

Getting the right amount of protein each day is crucial. If you eat too much protein, the process of gluconeogenesis will convert it into glucose, preventing ketosis. If you don't eat enough protein, the body can't maintain its muscles and cells. For sedentary or lightly active people, the right amount is 0.8 grams of protein per pound of lean body mass (that's weight of everything except body fat).

MACRO TIP • **Protein is typically 15 to 30 percent of total calorie intake on a keto diet.** For a rough estimate of how many grams of protein you need, divide your weight in pounds by 2. For example, if you weigh 180 pounds, your daily protein goal is approximately 90 grams per day.

3. USE FAT AS A LEVER

Don't fear fat! Fat is our source of energy as well as satiety. Your intake of carbs and protein stay constant each day on the keto diet, but fat is a lever you can pull up or down to gain or lose weight. So if your goal is weight loss, eat enough fat to be satisfied (and you'll still get plenty!), but there's no need to "get your fats in" past that.

FOODS TO EAT:

- **Healthy fats** like avocados, avocado oil, butter, and coconut oil

- **Leafy greens** like lettuce, spinach, and kale

- **Low carb vegetables** that grow above-ground, like zucchini, cauliflower, and asparagus

- **Meat** like beef and pork

- **Poultry** like chicken and turkey

- **Seafood** like fish, shrimp, and crab

- **Full-fat dairy** like hard and soft cheeses, cream cheese, mascarpone, and heavy cream

- **Eggs**

- **Sugar-free beverages** like water, coffee, and tea

- **Herbs and spices** like basil, dill, cumin, and cinnamon

- **Low carb condiments** like mayonnaise, hot sauce, and mustard

FOODS TO AVOID:

- **Grains**—including wheat of any kind, bread, pasta, rice, oats, cereal, corn, etc.

- **Sugar**—including table sugar, candy, pastries, cakes, ice cream, chocolate, soda, juice, honey, maple syrup, etc.

- **Starchy vegetables**—including potatoes, sweet potatoes, parsnips, etc.

- **Legumes**—including beans, lentils, chickpeas, etc. (Peanuts are an exception in moderation.)

- **High-sugar fruits**—including bananas, pineapples, oranges, apples, grapes, etc.

- **Low-fat dairy products**—including cow's milk and cheese; **all full-fat cow's milk**—except heavy cream

- **Seed and vegetable oils**—especially margarine, canola oil, corn oil, grapeseed oil, and soybean oil

- **Processed "low carb" foods** like packaged cookies, ice cream bars, or low carb wheat tortillas—this depends on ingredients, so read labels for hidden sugar, starch, and artificial ingredients

FOODS TO ENJOY IN MODERATION:

- **Low carb fruit** like raspberries and blueberries

- **Nuts and seeds** like almonds, macadamia nuts, and sunflower seeds

- **Sugar-free sweeteners** like erythritol, monk fruit, and stevia

- **Low carb flours** like almond flour, coconut flour, and flaxseed meal

Get a full list of keto foods with net carb counts at www.wholesomeyum.com/low-carb-keto-food-list

4. DRINK LOTS OF WATER

Water is always a good thing, but especially
on a keto diet. When you eat carbohydrates,
your body stores the extra as glycogen in
the liver, where they are bound to water
molecules. A state of ketosis depletes this
glycogen, which allows you to burn fat—but
it also means you are storing less water,
making it easier to get dehydrated. Instead
of the traditional recommendation of 8 cups
of water per day, aim for 16 cups.

5. KEEP UP ELECTROLYTES

The major electrolytes in our bodies
are sodium, potassium, and magnesium.
Because a low carb diet (especially a keto
diet!) reduces the amount of water you
store, this can flush out electrolytes and
make you feel sick (called "keto flu"). This is
temporary, but you can avoid or eliminate it
by salting your food liberally, drinking broth,
and eating pickled vegetables. Some people
also choose to take supplements for electrolytes, but it's best to first consult a doctor.

6. EAT ONLY WHEN YOU ARE HUNGRY

Get out of the mindset that you need to eat
four to six meals per day or constantly snack.
Eating too frequently on a keto diet is not
necessary, and can affect weight loss. Eat
when you're hungry, but if you aren't, don't.
Eating fewer carbs will make this much easier, as it naturally suppresses appetite.

7. FOCUS ON WHOLE FOODS

Eating natural or whole foods is not required
to restrict carbohydrates, but eating processed foods on a keto diet will not make it
easy to get rid of those junk food cravings,
and it's certainly not good for your body. The
keto lifestyle is about getting healthier, and
that means dropping processed food.

STOCKING YOUR KETO PANTRY

Stocking your keto pantry is one of the highest impact things you can do before you start the keto lifestyle and begin making the recipes in this book. It will be much easier to stay on track if you are prepared with ingredients on hand that support this lifestyle.

LOW CARB FLOURS AND BAKING

- **Blanched almond flour**—Almond flour is my go-to replacement for white flour in recipes, but in some ways it does work differently since it doesn't have the binding properties of gluten. Make sure it's blanched and finely ground! The ones that look speckled or are labeled "almond meal" won't work well for most baking applications.

- **Coconut flour**—Coconut flour is extremely absorbent and doesn't work like any other flour. It's fussy and requires special recipes developed specifically for it. Don't try to replace coconut flour with something else, or replace another ingredient in a recipe with coconut flour. One of the most common misconceptions is that almond flour and coconut flour are interchangeable, but they are *not*!

- **Flaxseed meal**—A great nut-free option for baking, plus it provides fiber and helps baked goods stay together. Any kind will do, but I recommend golden for the best flavor.

- **Psyllium husk powder**—This works great to give low carb baked goods a chewy quality, plus it provides a ton of fiber.

- **Sunflower seed meal**—Definitely not a requirement, but this can be a good almond flour substitute if you or your family has a nut allergy.

- **Xanthan gum**—This can be used as a thickener for sauces, dressings, and soups, or as a binder for baked goods.

- **Gelatin powder**—Another ingredient used as a thickener or binder. It also has the benefit of providing collagen protein!

- **Cocoa powder**—Make sure it's unsweetened!

- **Unsweetened baking chocolate**—This often comes in baker's chocolate bars.

- **Sugar-free chocolate chips**—Look for ones sweetened with stevia instead of maltitol.

SUGAR-FREE SWEETENERS

I recommend only *natural* sugar-free sweeteners. Here are the best ones:

- **Erythritol:** My favorite sweetener, used for most recipes in this book! Erythritol tastes great, does not get metabolized, and rarely causes digestive issues unlike other sugar alcohols. It's about 70 percent as sweet as sugar. Just like sugar, erythritol can come in granulated or powdered forms, and granulated is assumed when not specified. Powdered erythritol is simply erythritol that has been ground to a fine powder, the consistency of powdered sugar.

- **Xylitol:** An alternative to erythritol. It tastes great, measures 1:1 like sugar, and has benefits for the teeth, but may cause stomach upset in large quantities and is fatal to dogs.

- **Monk fruit:** Monk fruit is very concentrated and expensive on its own. I prefer to buy a monk fruit/erythritol blend that measures 1:1 like sugar, which you'll also see in this book.

- **Stevia:** Like monk fruit, stevia is also very concentrated and easiest to use in a blend with a bulking agent like erythritol. Stevia has an aftertaste that many people dislike, but it is a great option if you don't mind it.

There are dozens of sweetener brands out there—and I even have my own Wholesome Yum brand sweeteners! Many of them are blends with different ratios, even if the name sometimes implies it isn't a blend. Always read ingredients for various fillers and check how a sweetener measures compared to sugar. Sweeteners not only provide sweetness but also create bulk and affect the wet/dry ratio of a recipe, so use caution when substituting sweeteners that have drastically different volumes or consistencies.

For the recipes in this book, you'll see granulated erythritol or a 1:1 monk fruit/erythritol blend. For uses that need a smooth consistency, such as frostings, sauces, dressings, or cheesecake, use a powdered sweetener so that you don't get a gritty result. (Sugar-free sweeteners do not dissolve as well as sugar and generally don't caramelize at all.)

> To learn more about sweeteners and learn how to substitute them, check out the guide and conversion calculator at
>
> www.wholesomeyum.com/sweeteners

HEALTHY FATS

- **Avocado oil**
- **Butter**—grass-fed is more beneficial, but not required
- **Coconut oil**
- **Ghee**
- **MCT oil**
- **Olive oil**

CONDIMENTS

You can easily make your own keto-friendly condiments—there are several in this book! However, for convenience you may want to buy some of them. Condiments are notorious for containing hidden sugars, starches, and artificial ingredients, so read labels carefully.

- **Coconut aminos**
- **Fish sauce**
- **Horseradish**
- **Hot sauce**
- **Lemon and lime juice**
- **Marinara sauce**
- **Mayonnaise**
- **Mustard**
- **Salsa**
- **Sugar-free salad dressing:** Creamy or olive oil–based. Avoid seed oils, like soybean or canola.
- **Vinegar:** White, apple cider, balsamic, white wine, red wine, etc.

MISCELLANEOUS

- **Dried herbs:** Basil, dill, rosemary, thyme, bay leaves, etc.
- **Extracts:** Vanilla extract, real maple extract, almond extract, etc. Make sure these are natural and have no sugar added!
- **Nuts and seeds:** Almonds, macadamia nuts, pecans, sunflower seeds, etc.
- **Nut butter:** Almond butter and peanut butter are the most common, but any nut butter without added sugar is great.
- **Pork rinds:** Great for snacking, but you can also crush them to use as a substitute for breadcrumbs.
- **Spices:** Salt, black pepper, cumin, paprika, garlic powder, ground ginger, etc.

For a list of specific brands I recommend, check out my Shop page at

www.wholesomeyum.com/shop

Soon, you'll be able to purchase my own keto-friendly flours, sweeteners, and even ready-made keto pizza!

THE ULTIMATE GUIDE TO FATHEAD DOUGH

I'm devoting a special section of this book to fathead dough, for two good reasons:

1. It's amazing! Seriously, if you love bread and baked goods, this dough will become a lifesaver. I have yet to find anyone who doesn't like it—keto or not!

2. It can be a little challenging to work with at first, especially if you are used to baking with regular flour. It acts and works very differently, and can take some practice. So I'm going to walk you through it step by step. It's so worth it, I promise!

This section will tell you *everything* you need to know about this amazing keto dough! From the various ways to make it to the best tips to perfecting it, I highly recommend reading this guide before you make your first batch.

WHAT IS FATHEAD DOUGH?

Fathead dough started out as a recipe for low carb pizza crust, but it can be used for many things! The basic ingredients are mozzarella cheese, cream cheese, eggs, and some type of low carb flour, typically almond or coconut.

The main appeal of this dough is that it turns out chewy like real pizza or bread does, which is often challenging with other low carb baked goods. I've served recipes with fathead dough to my non-keto extended family and friends hundreds of times, and every time they are a hit!

The original recipe came from a 2009 documentary called *Fat Head*, which is where the dough got its name. That version was made with almond flour. I have adapted it with some different methods, a coconut flour version, and variations for different uses.

BEST USES FOR FATHEAD DOUGH

The best feature of fathead dough is its chewiness, though it also gets crispy when baked thin. The texture makes it perfect for dense and chewy baked goods such as pizza, calzones, tortillas, bagels, flatbreads, dumplings, rolls, etc.

Another advantage over other low carb doughs is that it's pliable. This makes it great for recipes where the dough needs to bend or wrap.

Fathead dough is not suitable for baked goods that need to be crumbly, light, or airy, such as cakes, muffins, and the like.

BASIC FATHEAD DOUGH RECIPE INGREDIENTS

You can make fathead dough with almond flour or coconut flour. Below are the basic ingredients for each version. There are also some common ingredient variations used for some recipes.

INGREDIENTS FOR ALMOND FLOUR VERSION

- 1½ *cups (6 ounces)* **shredded mozzarella cheese**
- 1 *ounce (2 tablespoons)* **cream cheese, cut into cubes**
- 1 *large* **egg, whisked**
- ¾ *cup (3 ounces)* **finely ground blanched almond flour**

INGREDIENTS FOR COCONUT FLOUR VERSION

- 1½ *cups (6 ounces)* **shredded mozzarella cheese**
- 1 *ounce (2 tablespoons)* **cream cheese, cut into cubes**
- 2 *large* **eggs, whisked**
- ⅓ *cup (1.3 ounces)* **coconut flour**

INGREDIENT VARIATIONS

In addition to the above ingredient templates, you can add or remove ingredients as shown below. For recipes in this book that use fathead dough, it will be specified in that recipe's ingredient list what adjustments to the dough, if any, are required.

- **Fathead dough without cream cheese**
  Simply skip the cream cheese and melt the mozzarella alone. This makes sturdier dough that is easier to bend, such as for tortillas. (See Pliable Fathead Tortillas, page 201.)

- **Fathead dough with baking powder**
  Add ½ tablespoon baking powder at the same time as the flour (if making a double batch of the dough, add 1 tablespoon). This is used for recipes where you want the fathead dough to rise a bit. (See Fathead Gnocchi, page 150; Chewy Fathead Bagels, page 189; and Italian Garlic Bread Sticks, page 198.)

  I did not include baking powder in the pizza crust recipes in this book (I like a thin, crispy crust!), but you easily could if you are making a thicker crust and want some lift.

- **Fathead dough with sweetener**
  Add 2 tablespoons erythritol, or other sweetener of choice, at the same time as the flour (if making a double batch of dough, use ¼ cup). This is used for recipes that are sweet. (See Cinnamon Roll Dessert Pizza, page 223.)

  Note that you can't add too much sweetener, as this will disrupt the consistency of the dough, but 2 tablespoons per batch works. The sweet version of the dough may be stickier to work with than the regular kind—check the tips section on how to remedy that.

HOW TO MAKE THE DOUGH

There are three basic steps to prepare fat-head dough: (1) melt the cheeses, (2) knead the dough, and (3) use the dough as called for in your recipe. Each step has a couple of methods you can use. I'll cover all of them below and you can choose the methods you prefer.

STEP 1: MELT THE CHEESES TOGETHER

MICROWAVE METHOD:

1. Combine the shredded mozzarella and cubed cream cheese in a large bowl.
2. Microwave for about 90 seconds, stirring halfway through, until smooth and easy to stir. Stir again at the end to make it uniform.

STOVETOP METHOD:

1. In a double boiler, combine the shredded mozzarella and cubed cream cheese.
2. Heat for a few minutes, stirring occasionally, until smooth, easy to stir, and uniform.
   See Figure 1 for the melted cheese.

STEP 2: KNEAD THE DOUGH

BY HAND METHOD:

1. If the recipe requires baking powder and/or sweetener, stir these with the flour in a small bowl. (Skip this step if making the original recipe without modifications.)
2. Stir the beaten egg(s) and flour (or flour mixture) into the cheeses in a large bowl.

3. Knead with your hands and squeeze rapidly through your fingers, until a uniform dough forms.

FOOD PROCESSOR OR STAND MIXER METHOD:

1. Add the flour to a food processor fitted with either the metal blade or a dough blade, or a stand mixer fitted with a dough hook. If the recipe requires baking powder and/or sweetener, add them as well and turn on the machine to mix together.
2. Add the egg(s). Turn on the food processor or stand mixer again to mix.
3. Add the melted cheese mixture (make sure it's still hot enough to be easy to stir) and position the blade or dough hook in the center of the cheese. Turn on the food processor or mixer again and keep it running until a uniform dough forms. (You may need to stop to scrape any flour left on the sides or bottom away from the blade or dough hook.)
   See Figure 2 for the dough.

STEP 3: MAKE THE RECIPE AND BAKE

Once the dough has come together and is uniform, you can follow the recipe as directed to form it into the shape you need and bake it. However, if it's too sticky or can't be formed into a ball (Figure 3), you may need to chill it, use oiled hands to work with it, or both. See the tips on the following pages.

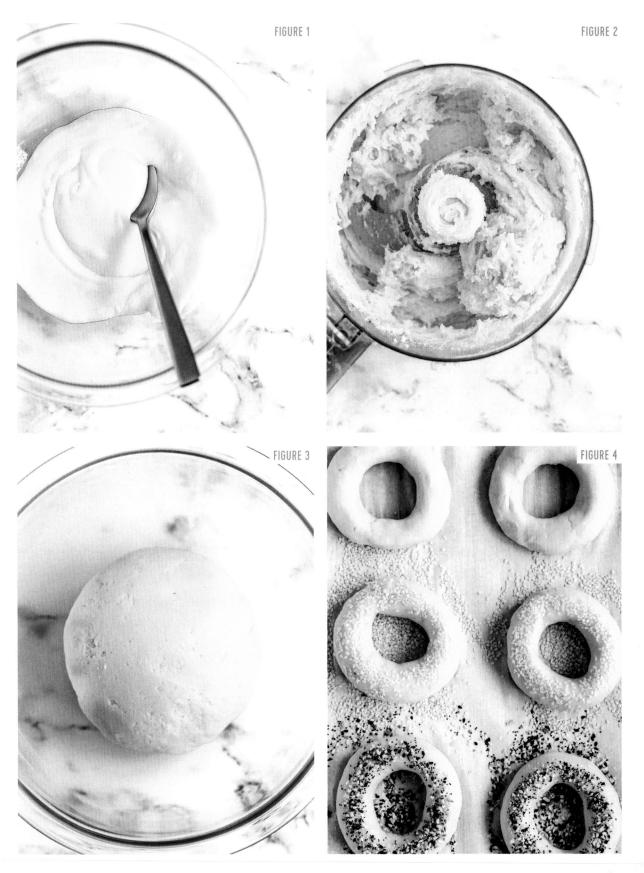

FIGURE 1

FIGURE 2

FIGURE 3

FIGURE 4

HOW TO DOUBLE THE RECIPE

Some of the recipes in this book that call for fathead dough, such as bagels, require doubling the dough recipe (the ingredient list will call for "double recipe Fathead Dough").

In this case, simply double the amounts listed (including the amounts of baking powder or sweetener if using) and follow the same instructions. It may take longer to melt the cheeses together in the first step.

TIPS FOR WORKING WITH FATHEAD DOUGH

Once you get the method down for making fathead dough, it's one of the easiest recipes ever! However, here are tips to help you nail it right away and troubleshoot any potential issues:

GET THE RIGHT INGREDIENTS

The fathead dough recipe uses pretty common ingredients, but here are two that come in different types where the right type is important:

- **Mozzarella:** Make sure the mozzarella is the firm, hard mozzarella. You can buy it preshredded or shred it yourself. Just avoid the soft, bright white fresh mozzarella that comes in a ball, as this has too much moisture content.

- **Almond flour:** If you make the almond flour version of the fathead dough, be sure to use finely ground blanched almond flour. Your fathead dough may be gritty if you use almond meal or ground almonds, or if your almond flour looks speckled. You want a super-finely ground almond flour that is uniformly ivory in color.

MAKE SURE THE DOUGH IS UNIFORM IN APPEARANCE

It's important for the dough to thoroughly mix together, so that it's uniform in appearance and texture. You shouldn't see any separate clumps of cheese or flour in the final result.

If you have trouble getting your ingredients to incorporate, it could be that the cheese solidified too quickly after melting, before mixing with the flour and egg. It will only mix well if it's soft and easy to stir.

There's a solution if your cheese solidified too fast and the dough doesn't want to come together. Simply reheat the dough slightly, about 30 seconds in the microwave or maybe a bit longer in a double boiler—just enough to soften the dough a bit. Be careful not to heat the dough for too long to avoid actually cooking it. Once it heats up a bit, it should be easier to knead again (regardless of which method you are using).

CHILL THE DOUGH IF NEEDED

After the fathead dough comes together, sometimes it can be too sticky to shape or roll out for your recipe, or it can look super mushy, almost like mashed potatoes. (This is most common if your kitchen is on the warmer side, and the coconut flour version is more prone to it compared to almond flour.)

If this happens, chill the dough in the refrigerator for 15 to 30 minutes, until it's slightly cool to the touch, but not frigid cold. It should be soft and fairly similar in consistency to dough typically made with wheat flour.

Note that chilling for too long can make the dough very stiff, which would make it challenging to bend or roll out as well. If you let it get too cold, bring it back to room temperature on the counter.

USE OILED HANDS WHEN FORMING THE DOUGH INTO SHAPES

This is not always required, but it can be a huge help. If your dough is too sticky even after chilling, wash your hands and cover them in a neutral-tasting oil, like avocado oil.

Using oiled hands as you shape or roll it for your recipe will prevent it from sticking to your hands. For cases where you roll it between parchment paper, you can also oil the parchment paper so that it doesn't stick, either.

MAKING FATHEAD DOUGH AHEAD OF TIME

Preparing fathead dough ahead of time is a huge timesaver! Here are several options to do so:

- **Make the dough to store in the fridge.** You can make a ball of dough, wrap it in plastic to prevent drying out, and refrigerate it for up to several days. It may be stiff when you take it out, so let it warm up at room temperature, until it's slightly cool yet soft.

- **Freeze the dough.** You can freeze a ball of dough if you want to store it long term. It will keep for months in the freezer, tightly wrapped to avoid drying out or freezer burn. Before using, simply thaw the dough in the fridge for 24 hours, then let it come to slightly cooler than room temperature on the counter.

- **Refrigerate or freeze prebaked dough.** This is the most convenient option, and the one I recommend most! You can easily prebake a pizza crust, bagels, tortillas, and more. Keep the baked goods in the refrigerator or freeze until ready to use. For most uses, you can reheat them straight from the freezer. (For example, pop frozen fathead bagels in the toaster, or top a frozen crust with toppings and bake.)

SAMPLE EASY KETO MEAL PLAN

To get you started, below is a sample keto meal plan using recipes from this book. It's designed to save you time by taking advantage of meal prep and occasional leftovers.

This plan approximately fits typical keto macros, with each day under 25 grams net carbs. Your individual macro needs will vary based on your weight, gender, health goals, and other factors. You can fill in the rest of your macro needs with snacks or by adjusting portion sizes if needed.

	BREAKFAST	LUNCH	DINNER
MONDAY	MEAL PREP: **Sheet Pan Sausage Breakfast Sandwich (page 49)** 552 calories 3 g net carbs 46 g fat 28 g protein	MEAL PREP: **Taco-Stuffed Avocado (page 65)** 413 calories 4 g net carbs 33 g fat 20 g protein	**Kielbasa Veggie Sheet Pan Dinner (page 115)** 686 calories 7 g net carbs 59 g fat 26 g protein
TUESDAY	**Double-Berry Smoothie (page 33)** 256 calories 11 g net carbs 18 g fat 8 g protein	MEAL PREP: **Sun-Dried Tomato and Arugula Avocado Toast (page 74)** 453 calories 9 g net carbs 38 g fat 10 g protein	**Maple Pecan-Crusted Salmon (page 121) + Lemon-Garlic Roasted Broccoli (page 154)** 501 calories 4 g net carbs 41 g fat 26 g protein
WEDNESDAY	MEAL PREP: **Sheet Pan Sausage Breakfast Sandwich (page 49)** 552 calories 3 g net carbs 46 g fat 28 g protein	LEFTOVERS: **Kielbasa Veggie Sheet Pan Dinner (page 115)** 686 calories 7 g net carbs 59 g fat 26 g protein	**15-Minute Egg Roll in a Bowl (page 100)** 231 calories (double serving if desired) 4 g net carbs 15 g fat 15 g protein

	BREAKFAST	LUNCH	DINNER
THURSDAY	Double-Berry Smoothie (page 33) 256 calories 11 g net carbs 18 g fat 8 g protein	MEAL PREP: Taco Stuffed Avocado (page 65) 413 calories 4 g net carbs 33 g fat 20 g protein	Tuscan Garlic Chicken Casserole (page 104) 430 calories 8 g net carbs 29 g fat 32 g protein
FRIDAY	MEAL PREP: Sheet Pan Sausage Breakfast Sandwich (page 49) 552 calories 3 g net carbs 46 g fat 28 g protein	LEFTOVERS: Tuscan Garlic Chicken Casserole (page 104) 430 calories 8 g net carbs 29 g fat 32 g protein	Crispy Orange Chicken (page 129) + Cauliflower Fried Rice (page 145) 434 calories 13 g net carbs 24 g fat 34 g protein
SATURDAY	Flourless Chocolate Chip Peanut Butter Waffles (page 37) 387 calories 7 g net carbs 31 g fat 17 g protein	MEAL PREP: Sun-Dried Tomato and Arugula Avocado Toast (page 74) 453 calories 9 g net carbs 38 g fat 10 g protein	Fathead Pizza Crust (page 99): 2 slices with sugar-free marinara, mozzarella, and toppings of choice 288 calories* 4 g net carbs 24 g fat 16 g protein
SUNDAY	Spicy Mediterranean Shakshuka (page 55) 248 calories 8 g net carbs 15 g fat 16 g protein	Honey-Mustard Chicken Cobb Salad (page 91) 336 calories 5 g net carbs 29 g fat 19 g protein	Chili-Lime Turkey Burgers (page 136) + Almond Flax Burger Buns (page 207) 686 calories 7 g net carbs 55 g fat 37 g protein

* Nutrition info for pizza does not include toppings, which will vary based on what you add. This should be enough for a meal after adding toppings.

PREP INSTRUCTIONS →

BREAKFAST MEAL PREP INSTRUCTIONS

- **Sheet Pan Sausage Breakfast Sandwich**—Prepare and assemble the sandwiches. Wrap individually. Refrigerate the portions for the week and freeze the rest. Heat the day of.

LUNCH MEAL PREP INSTRUCTIONS

- **Taco Stuffed Avocado**—Brown the beef and chop the fillings. Assemble the day of.
- **Sun-Dried Tomato and Arugula Avocado Toast**—Make The Best 90-Second Bread (page 194). On the day of, toast the bread, mash the avocado, and add the toppings.

DINNER MEAL PREP INSTRUCTIONS (OPTIONAL)

You don't have to do these ahead, but doing so can make dinner prep faster on the day of. I recommend doing this as batch prep on Sunday for the week ahead!

- **Kielbasa Veggie Sheet Pan Dinner**—Slice the kielbasa and chop the veggies.
- **Maple Pecan-Crusted Salmon**—Chop the pecans and prepare the pecan topping.
- **Lemon-Garlic Roasted Broccoli**—Chop the broccoli.

- **15-Minute Egg Roll in a Bowl**—Shred the cabbage, or to save time, just buy coleslaw mix.
- **Tuscan Garlic Chicken Casserole**—Assemble the casserole ahead and store in the fridge. Bake the day of.
- **Fathead Pizza Crust**—Prebake the crust. Refrigerate or freeze. The day of, add sauce and toppings, and bake.
- **Chili-Lime Turkey Burgers**—Make the Almond Flax Burger Buns.

MORE WEEKLY KETO MEAL PLANS

For more weekly plans like this one, plus loads of time-saving and meal prep tips, sign up for Wholesome Yum Weekly Meal Plans at: www.wholesomeyum.com/low-carb-keto-meal-plan. Soon you'll also be able to customize your meal plans to your preferences!

KETO SWAPS FOR YOUR FAVORITE FOODS ➡

One of my favorite things in the world is showing people that a keto lifestyle does not have to be restrictive or boring! You can easily replace all your favorite foods with keto versions.

Check out these healthy keto swaps for some of your favorite comfort foods!

KETO SWAPS FOR YOUR FAVORITE FOODS

CRAVING THIS?	HAVE THIS KETO VERSION INSTEAD!
Bagels	Chewy Fathead Bagels (page 189)
Bread	Easy All-Purpose Bread (page 197), Italian Garlic Bread Sticks (page 198), The Best 90-Second Bread (page 194)
Brownies	Fudgy Brownies (page 216)
Burger	Chili-Lime Turkey Burgers (page 136) on Almond Flax Burger Buns (page 207)
Cereal with milk	Cinnamon Crunch Cereal (page 34)
Cheesecake	Classic Cheesecake (page 210)
Chicken tenders	Crispy Chicken Tenders (page 66)
Chili	Classic Hearty Beef Chili (page 83)
Coffee cake	Coffee Cake Zucchini Bread (page 203)
Crackers	3-Ingredient Almond Flour Crackers (page 163)
French fries	Crispy Avocado Fries with Chipotle Dip (page 175)
Ice cream	Hazelnut Ice Cream (page 224)
Latte	Butter Coffee Latte (page 30)
Lasagna	Lazy Lasagna Chicken (page 70)
Mashed potatoes	Loaded Cauliflower Mash (page 149)
Muffins	Blueberry Muffins (page 215), Carrot Cake Muffins (page 228)
Nachos	Mini Bell Pepper Nachos (page 107)
Onion rings	Crispy Bacon Wrapped Onion Rings (page 167)
Pancakes	Almond Flour Pancakes (page 29), Pumpkin Coconut Flour Pancakes (page 38)
Pasta	Spaghetti Squash Bolognese (page 108), Almond Pesto Zucchini Noodles (page 158)
Pizza	Fathead Pizza Crust (page 99) with pizza toppings
Potato chips	Easy Baked Zucchini Chips (page 164)
Potato salad	Cauliflower "Potato" Salad (page 80)
Rice	Cauliflower Fried Rice (page 145)
Tacos	Pan-Fried Baja Fish Tacos (page 116), Cheese Taco Shells (page 193) with taco fillings, Taco-Stuffed Avocado (page 65)
Tortillas/wraps	Pliable Fathead Tortillas (page 201), Thai Beef Lettuce Wraps (page 69)

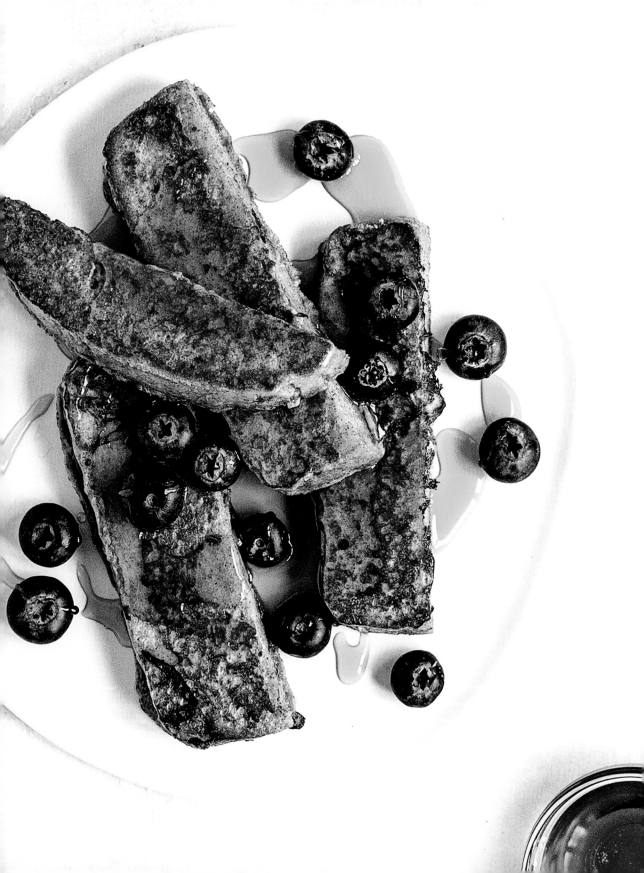

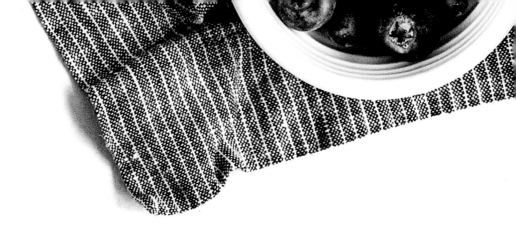

SWEET BREAKFASTS

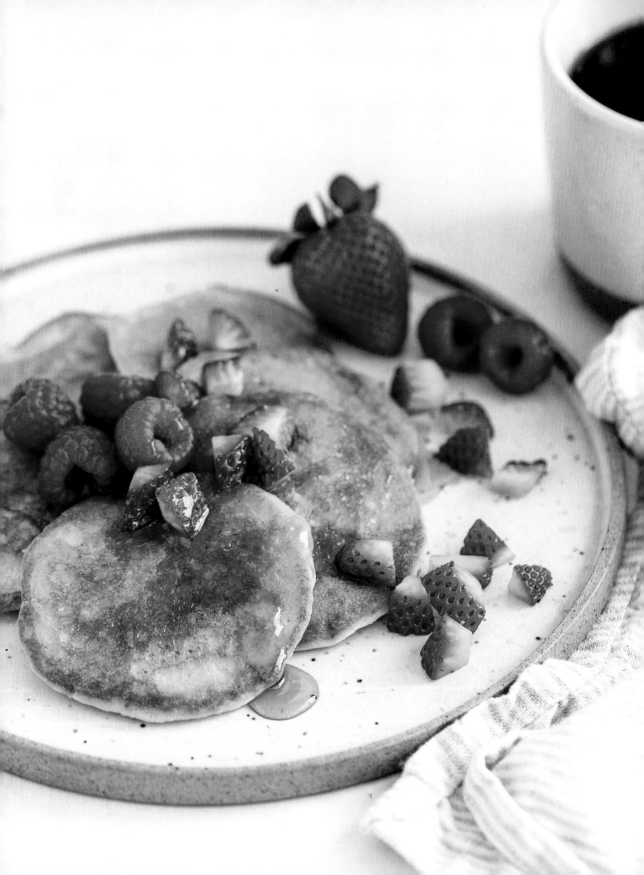

ALMOND FLOUR PANCAKES

I've made a copious amount of low carb pancakes over the years but keep coming back to these almond flour pancakes more than any other recipe. They are now synonymous with lazy weekend mornings spent with my family! And they taste so good, they're just the thing to win over *your* family if they are on the fence about keto.

1. In a blender, combine all ingredients and blend until smooth. Let the batter rest for 5 to 10 minutes.

2. Preheat a large, very lightly oiled skillet over medium-low heat. (Keep oil very minimal for perfectly round pancakes.) Working in batches, pour circles of batter onto the pan, 2 tablespoons (⅛ cup) at a time for 3-inch pancakes. Cook 1½ to 2 minutes, until bubbles start to form on the edges. Flip and cook another minute or two, until browned on the other side.

3. Repeat with the remaining batter.

2 cups (8 ounces) blanched almond flour

¼ cup erythritol

1 tablespoon baking powder

¼ teaspoon sea salt

4 large eggs

⅔ cup unsweetened almond milk

¼ cup avocado oil, plus more for frying

2 teaspoons vanilla extract

MAKES 6 SERVINGS

SERVING SIZE
four 3-inch pancakes
(3.5 ounces total)

PER SERVING
355 calories
31 g fat
12 g total carbs
5 g net carbs
12 g protein

TIPS & VARIATIONS • Feel free to add your favorite add-ins, like blueberries, nuts, or chocolate chips.

• Any neutral-tasting fat, such as melted butter or liquid coconut oil, will work instead of avocado oil.

• If you have any trouble flipping the pancakes, covering with a lid during cooking can make it easier.

• Serve with Homemade Sugar-Free Maple Syrup (page 247) or sugar-free Raspberry Sauce (page 244).

• You can make the pancakes ahead and refrigerate or freeze them. To freeze, place in the freezer in a single layer on parchment paper, then, once frozen, transfer the pancakes to a freezer bag.

BUTTER COFFEE LATTE

Adding butter to coffee might seem a little strange if you haven't done it before, but it was seriously life-changing for me! It keeps hunger at bay, boosts energy, and is frothy like a latte. The addition of vanilla almond milk in this recipe makes it even more like a true latte, without adding carbs.

1. *cup (8 ounces)* **brewed coffee**

½ *tablespoon* **unsalted butter**

½ *tablespoon* **MCT oil**

3 *tablespoons* **unsweetened vanilla almond milk**

MAKES 1 SERVING

1. In a blender, combine coffee, butter, MCT oil, and almond milk and blend until frothy. (Do not just stir the ingredients together. This will make your coffee oily, not frothy—yuck.)

2. Pour into a mug to serve.

SERVING SIZE
one 10-ounce cup

PER SERVING
119 calories
13 g fat
0 g total carbs
0 g net carbs
0 g protein

TIPS & VARIATIONS • For a richer cup, you can increase butter and MCT oil to 1 tablespoon each. You might need to reduce coffee by a tablespoon to make room.

• To avoid having to clean a blender, you can use a handheld milk frother instead. However, the blender does make a frothier, better-tasting coffee.

• For a nut-free version, use coconut milk instead of almond milk.

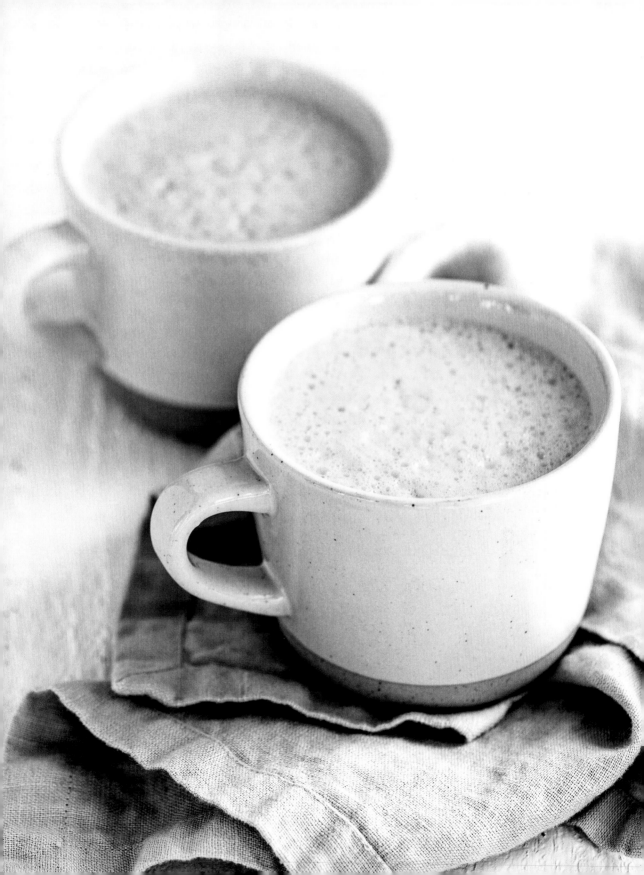

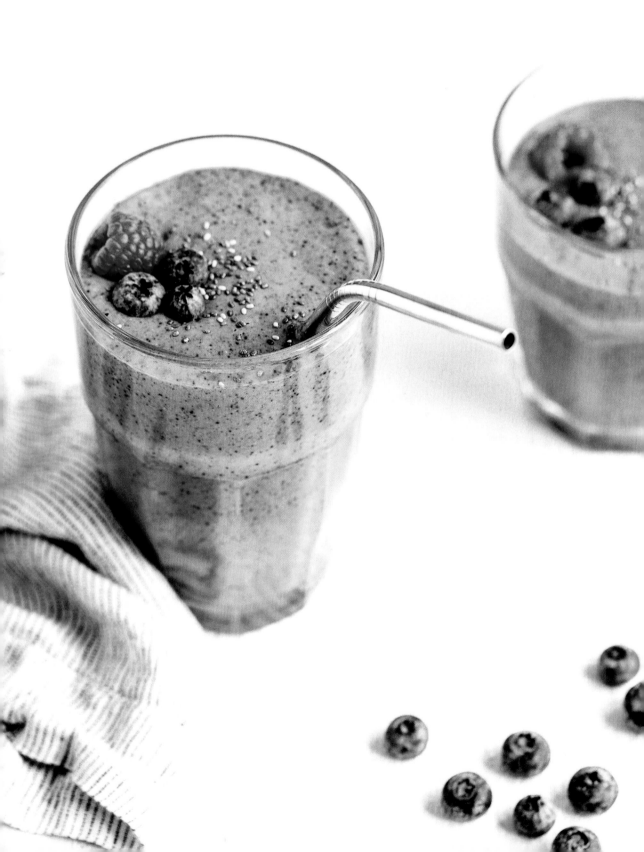

DOUBLE-BERRY SMOOTHIE

Smoothies are often touted as a health food, but most of them are loaded with sugar, either added to their ingredients or from tropical fruit. This low carb smoothie satisfies that fruit craving without you having to abandon your keto lifestyle.

In a blender, combine all the ingredients and blend until smooth. If using fresh berries, chill the smoothie for 30 minutes.

TIPS & VARIATIONS • If you want to bump up the fat content, you can increase the chia seeds. This will also make the smoothie thicker. For a thicker smoothie without changing the nutrition info, use frozen berries.

• Feel free to use any berries you like—raspberries, blueberries, blackberries, or strawberries. Raspberries (and blackberries) are the lowest in carbs and blueberries are the highest, so a combination balances them out.

• For a nut-free version, use coconut milk instead of almond milk.

• Any sugar-free sweetener you like will work! The amount will vary based on concentration, but it's easy to adjust to taste if using a different one.

2 cups unsweetened vanilla almond milk

2 cups (9 ounces) raspberries, fresh or frozen

1 cup (3.5 ounces) blueberries, fresh or frozen

½ cup monk fruit/ erythritol sweetener blend (1:1 sugar replacement)

½ cup almond butter, no sugar added

½ cup lemon juice

¼ cup chia seeds

MAKES 5 SERVINGS

SERVING SIZE
one 8-ounce cup

PER SERVING
256 calories
18 g fat
39 g total carbs
11 g net carbs
8 g protein

CINNAMON CRUNCH CEREAL

I have many childhood memories around food, but one of the most prominent is grabbing a big bowl of crunchy cinnamon cereal while I did my homework or watched TV after school. Since that cereal happens to be one of the most popular in America, I know I'm not the only one who misses it on the keto lifestyle. So I created this recipe for a homemade, keto-friendly version! I hope it conjures up some memories for you like it does for me every time.

1. Preheat the oven to 350°F.

2. In a large bowl, stir together the almond flour, erythritol, cinnamon, and sea salt.

3. In a small bowl, whisk together the eggs and vanilla. Add to the flour mixture and mix well until a dough forms.

4. Place the dough between two large greased pieces of parchment paper, at least 20 × 14 inches in size. Use a rolling pin to roll the dough out into a very thin rectangle, about ¹⁄₁₆ inch thick. It will tend to form an oval shape, so just rip off pieces and reattach to form a more angular shape. You can split the dough into two or more smaller batches if you can't get it to roll thin enough between your 20 × 14-inch pieces of parchment, or don't have a pan that large.

5. Place the bottom piece of parchment paper onto an extra-large baking sheet, at least 20 × 14 inches in size (or two 10 × 14-inch pans, if you've split your dough into smaller batches).

6. Cut the dough into ½-inch-wide strips. Rotate the pan 90 degrees and cut the dough strips into ½-inch-wide strips again, so you are left with ½-inch squares. You don't need to separate the squares; just cutting the dough is sufficient.

7. Transfer the pan(s) to the oven and bake for 8 to 12 minutes, until golden brown and crispy.

3½ cups (14 ounces) blanched almond flour

½ cup erythritol

2 teaspoons ground cinnamon

½ teaspoon sea salt

2 large eggs, beaten

1 teaspoon vanilla extract

CINNAMON COATING

½ cup erythritol

1 tablespoon ground cinnamon

2 tablespoons coconut oil, melted

MAKES 6 SERVINGS

SERVING SIZE
1 cup

PER SERVING
446 calories
39 g fat
26 g total carbs
7 g net carbs
16 g protein

8. **Meanwhile, make the cinnamon coating:** In a large zip-seal bag, combine the erythritol and cinnamon and shake to mix.

9. When the cereal is finished baking, remove from the oven and cool at room temperature to crisp up.

10. Brush the cereal on both sides with melted coconut oil. Then break apart the squares and add to the bag with the cinnamon-erythritol mixture. Shake to coat. Store in an airtight container in the pantry.

TIPS & VARIATIONS • If you prefer to save time or avoid a mess, you can mix the dough in a food processor.

• To make sure the cereal gets crunchy enough, roll out the dough evenly and uniformly, and bake until golden brown (baking time will vary significantly based on how thinly you roll out the dough). If the dough isn't rolled out evenly, some pieces may brown faster than others.

• Serve cinnamon crunch cereal with unsweetened almond milk or coconut milk.

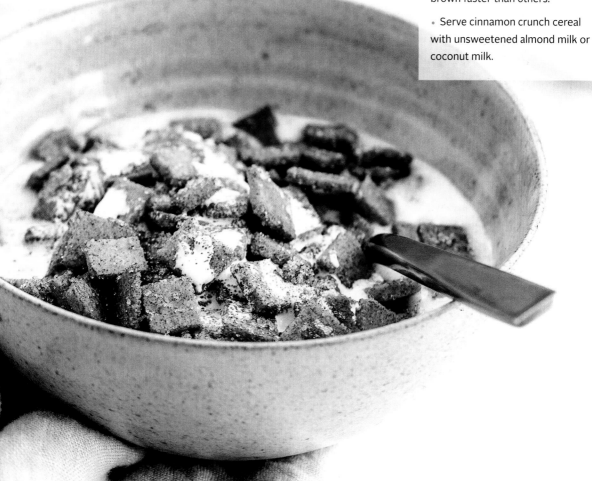

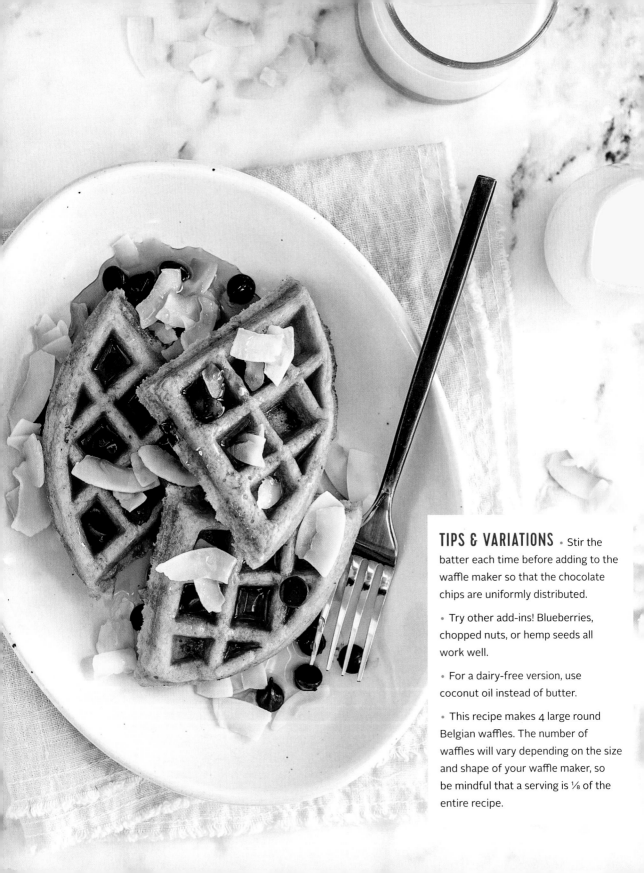

TIPS & VARIATIONS • Stir the batter each time before adding to the waffle maker so that the chocolate chips are uniformly distributed.

• Try other add-ins! Blueberries, chopped nuts, or hemp seeds all work well.

• For a dairy-free version, use coconut oil instead of butter.

• This recipe makes 4 large round Belgian waffles. The number of waffles will vary depending on the size and shape of your waffle maker, so be mindful that a serving is ⅛ of the entire recipe.

FLOURLESS CHOCOLATE CHIP PEANUT BUTTER WAFFLES

Flourless waffles are the perfect replacement for a familiar breakfast food. Peanut butter makes for waffles that are both light and crispy, without needing any specialty ingredients or even low carb flours. I love the chocolate chips, but if you choose to omit them, you can make this recipe on a whim with common pantry staples.

8 *large* eggs

1 *cup* peanut butter, no sugar added

¼ *cup* erythritol

4 *tablespoons (½ stick)* butter, melted

1 *teaspoon* baking powder

1 *teaspoon* vanilla extract

¾ *cup* sugar-free chocolate chips

MAKES 4 WAFFLES (8 SERVINGS)

1. In a large bowl, combine the eggs, peanut butter, erythritol, butter, baking powder, and vanilla. With an electric hand mixer, beat at medium speed until smooth.

2. Fold in the chocolate chips.

3. If you have time and want springier waffles, let the batter rest for 5 to 10 minutes.

4. Grease a Belgian waffle maker with butter or oil. Preheat according to the manufacturer's instructions.

5. Stir the batter, then immediately pour one-quarter of the batter evenly into the waffle maker. Cook according to the manufacturer's instructions. Usually, waffles are done when steam is no longer coming out, 4 to 5 minutes.

6. Repeat with the remaining batter to make 4 waffles total.

SERVING SIZE
½ large waffle (~2.3 ounces), or ⅛ of the recipe

PER SERVING
387 calories
31 g fat
15 g total carbs
7 g net carbs
17 g protein

PUMPKIN COCONUT FLOUR PANCAKES

I look forward to fall each year, and pumpkin is a big reason for that. But there are so many ways to use pumpkin beyond pumpkin pie—like pumpkin pancakes! In this recipe, coconut flour makes the perfect match for pumpkin puree: one thickens the batter and the other thins it out. The result? A delicious breakfast reminiscent of pumpkin pie except in pancake form.

1. In a blender, combine all the ingredients and puree until smooth.

2. Let the batter sit for 15 to 20 minutes to thicken and stabilize. (This will help with consistency and make the pancakes easier to flip.)

3. Heat an oiled skillet over medium heat. Working in batches, add 2 tablespoons (⅛ cup) batter for each pancake. Don't make them larger than 3 inches across, otherwise they will be hard to flip. Cover with a lid and when bubbles form on the edges, 1 to 2 minutes, flip and cook on the second side for 1 to 2 minutes.

4. Repeat with the remaining batter.

TIPS & VARIATIONS • Coconut flour can vary in absorbency by brand. If your batter is too thick or too thin after letting it sit for a couple of minutes, you can thin it out with a tiny bit more milk or thicken it with a tiny bit more coconut flour. If you make either of these additions, add just about a teaspoon at a time.

• Almond milk can be substituted for the coconut milk. Heavy cream works as well, if you are not dairy-free. Avoid regular dairy milk, which is high in carbs.

6 *large* eggs

½ *cup* canned unsweetened pumpkin puree

6 *tablespoons (1.5 ounces)* coconut flour

¼ *cup* unsweetened coconut milk

⅓ *cup* avocado oil

½ *cup* erythritol

1½ *tablespoons* pumpkin pie spice

1 *teaspoon* baking powder

1 *teaspoon* vanilla extract

MAKES 6 SERVINGS

SERVING SIZE
four 3-inch pancakes
(~4 ounces total)

PER SERVING
234 calories
18 g fat
12 g total carbs
4 g net carbs
8 g protein

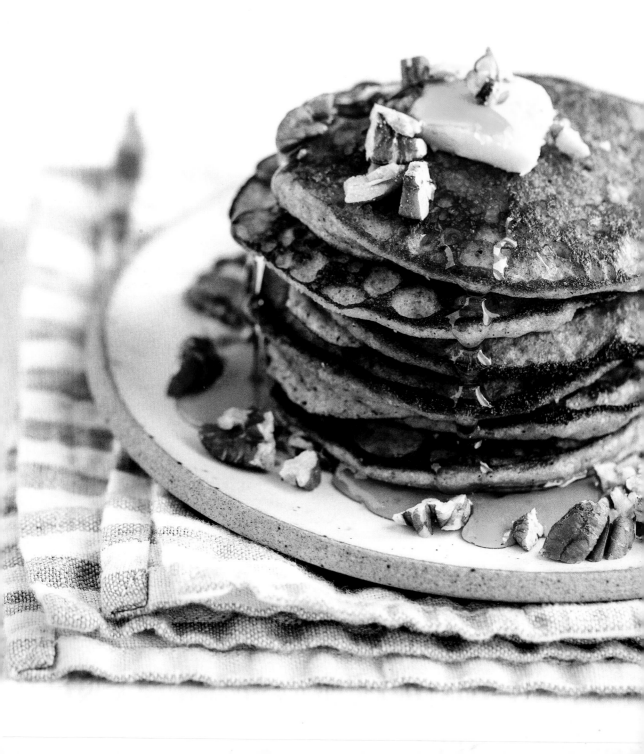

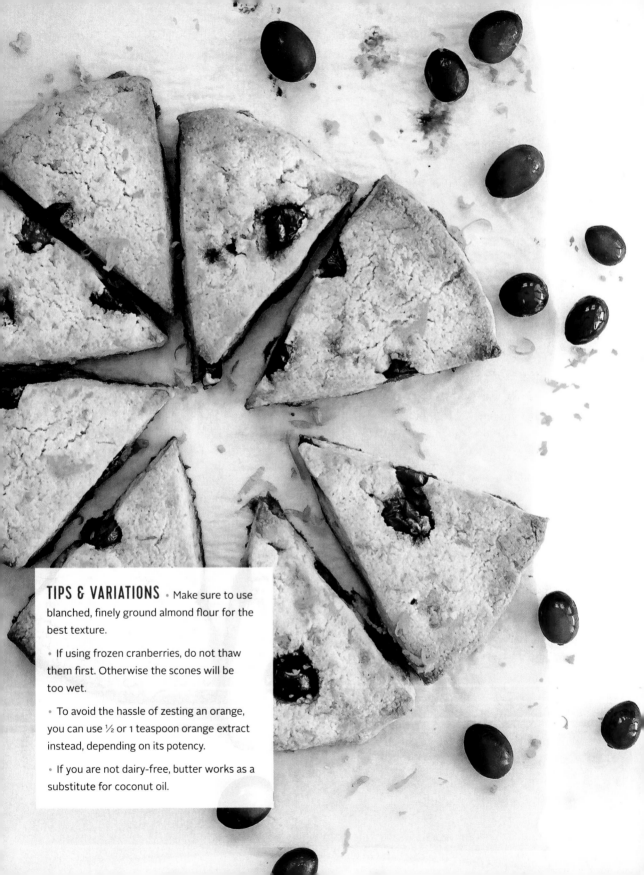

TIPS & VARIATIONS • Make sure to use blanched, finely ground almond flour for the best texture.

• If using frozen cranberries, do not thaw them first. Otherwise the scones will be too wet.

• To avoid the hassle of zesting an orange, you can use ½ or 1 teaspoon orange extract instead, depending on its potency.

• If you are not dairy-free, butter works as a substitute for coconut oil.

CRANBERRY-ORANGE SCONES

Before switching to a low carb lifestyle, one of my favorite pastimes was sitting in a coffee shop with my laptop or a friend, cradling a steaming latte and a scone. A lot has changed since then, but my love for scones sure hasn't! I hope these keto-friendly cranberry-orange scones will remind you of your favorite coffee shop, as they do for me, every time I make them.

1. Preheat the oven to 350°F. Line a baking sheet with parchment paper.

2. In a medium bowl, combine the almond flour, erythritol, baking powder, and sea salt.

3. In a small bowl, whisk together the melted coconut oil, orange zest, vanilla, and egg. Stir the wet mixture into the almond flour mixture, pressing with a spoon or spatula, until a uniform dough forms. (The dough should be pliable and dense, but not crumbly; add a little more coconut oil, a teaspoon at a time, if it's very dry.) Stir and press the cranberries into the dough.

4. Place the dough onto the lined pan and form a disc shape, about 1 inch thick and 6 inches in diameter. Cut into 8 wedges, like a pie or pizza. Move the pieces about 1 inch apart. Bake for 18 to 22 minutes, until golden.

5. Cool completely on the pan to firm up. (Scones will fall apart if you move them before cooling.)

2 cups (8 ounces) blanched almond flour

⅓ cup erythritol

½ teaspoon baking powder

¼ teaspoon sea salt

¼ cup coconut oil, melted

2 tablespoons orange zest

½ teaspoon vanilla extract

1 large egg

½ cup (2 ounces) cranberries, fresh or frozen

MAKES 8 SCONES

SERVING SIZE
one 3-inch scone (~2 ounces)

PER SERVING
232 calories
21 g fat
9 g total carbs
4 g net carbs
6 g protein

FRENCH TOAST STICKS

Making French toast sticks just brings me right back to my childhood! My mom and grandma used to make a savory version, without sugar. But when I started making my own, I found that I preferred the sweet version that Americans are accustomed to. Of course, these days I make mine low carb, using homemade low carb bread and sugar-free sweetener. And they are just as satisfying!

1. Stack the slices of bread and cut into thirds to create sticks (you'll have 18 sticks in total).

2. In a small bowl, whisk together the eggs, cream, sweetener, vanilla, cinnamon, and nutmeg.

3. Dip the bread sticks into the egg mixture, coating all sides and soak for a minute or two.

4. In a large skillet or griddle, heat 1 tablespoon of the butter over medium heat. Shake off the excess egg from the French toast sticks and immediately place onto the hot pan, without touching each other. Fry for 2 to 3 minutes on each side, until browned and crispy. Repeat with the remaining 1 tablespoon butter, bread sticks, and batter.

6 slices (½ inch thick) Easy All-Purpose Bread (page 197)

2 large eggs

3 tablespoons heavy cream

3 tablespoons monk fruit/erythritol sweetener blend (1:1 sugar replacement)

1 teaspoon vanilla extract

1 teaspoon ground cinnamon

⅛ teaspoon ground nutmeg

2 tablespoons butter, divided into 1 tablespoon and 1 tablespoon

MAKES 18 FRENCH TOAST STICKS (6 SERVINGS)

SERVING SIZE
3 French toast sticks (~2.8 ounces)

PER SERVING
292 calories
24 g fat
15 g total carbs
3 g net carbs
9 g protein

TIPS & VARIATIONS · Because low carb bread is less absorbent than regular wheat bread, thinner slices (about ½ inch thick) work best for keto French toast sticks.

· For flavor variations, add or substitute other extracts or spices, such as real maple extract or pumpkin pie spice, to the batter.

· For a dairy-free version, substitute coconut milk or almond milk for the heavy cream.

· Serve French Toast Sticks with Homemade Sugar-Free Maple Syrup (page 247), Raspberry Sauce (page 244), or butter.

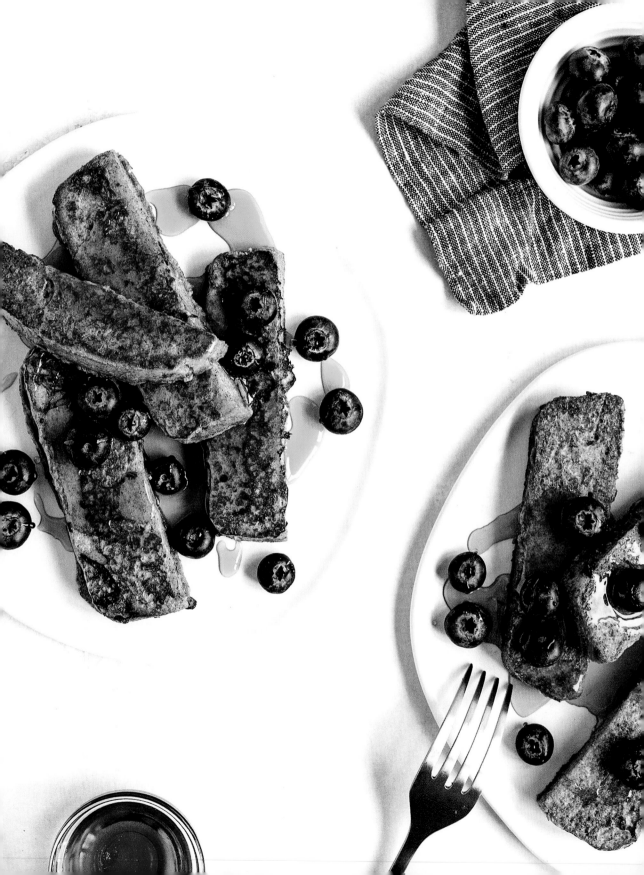

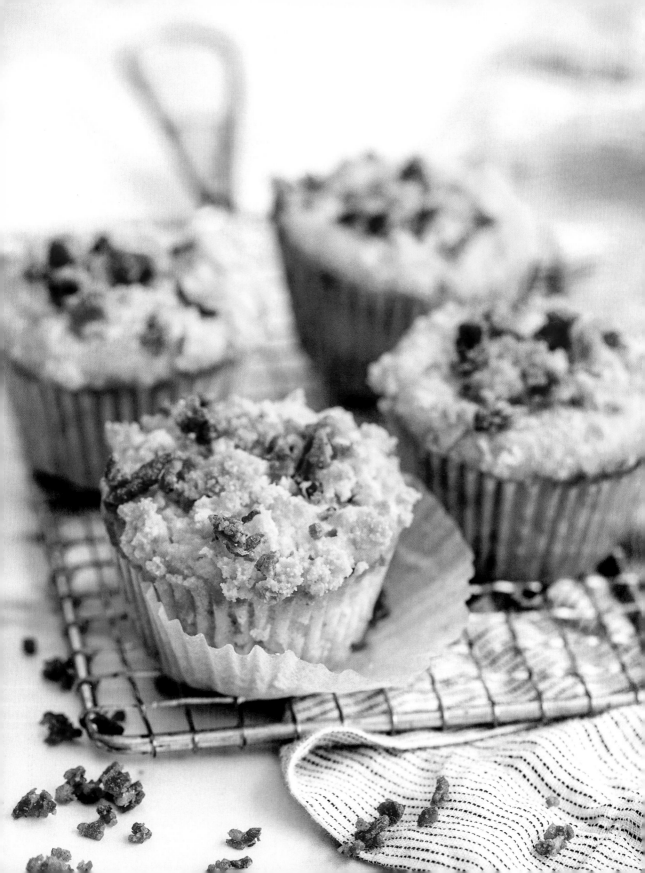

MAPLE-BACON PANCAKE MUFFINS

Maple syrup and bacon are a match made in heaven, but the combo doesn't usually conjure up the notion of muffins. Well, I say it should! Except we make ours low carb. These maple-bacon pancake muffins combine all the best things about pancakes and muffins, plus the bacon and loads of maple flavor take them over the top.

1. Preheat the oven to 350°F. Line 10 cups of a muffin tin with silicone or parchment paper muffin liners.

2. **Make the muffins:** In a large bowl, stir together the almond flour, erythritol, baking powder, and sea salt.

3. Mix in the melted butter, cream, eggs, and maple extract. Stir in the bacon bits.

4. Distribute the batter evenly among the muffin cups.

5. **Make the crumble topping:** In a small bowl, stir together the melted butter and maple extract. Add the almond flour, erythritol, and sea salt. Stir until uniform and crumbly. Sprinkle the crumble topping evenly over the muffins.

6. Bake for 25 to 30 minutes, until the tops of the muffins are golden and an inserted toothpick comes out clean.

MUFFINS

- 2½ cups (10 ounces) blanched almond flour
- ½ cup erythritol
- ½ tablespoon baking powder
- ¼ teaspoon sea salt
- 5 tablespoons + 1 teaspoon (⅔ stick) butter, melted
- ½ cup heavy cream
- 3 large eggs
- ½ teaspoon real maple extract
- ¾ cup cooked bacon bits

CRUMBLE TOPPING

- 1 tablespoon butter, melted
- ⅛ teaspoon real maple extract
- ⅓ cup (1.3 ounces) blanched almond flour
- 2 tablespoons erythritol
- Pinch of sea salt

MAKES 10 MUFFINS

TIPS & VARIATIONS · Make sure to use blanched, finely ground almond flour for the best texture.

· You can stretch the number of servings to 12 muffins if you want to reduce carbs and calories per muffin, but doing so will mean flatter muffin tops.

· For a dairy-free version, substitute coconut oil for the butter and coconut milk or almond milk for the heavy cream.

SERVING SIZE
1 muffin (~3 ounces)

PER SERVING
341 calories
30 g fat
11 g total carbs
4 g net carbs
12 g protein

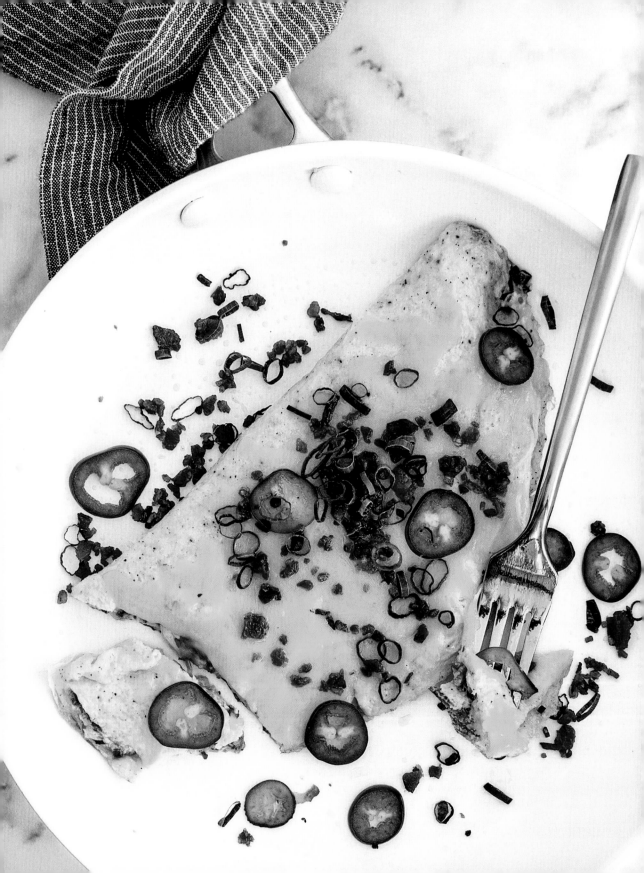

SAVORY BREAKFASTS

JALAPEÑO POPPER STUFFED OMELET

An omelet is one of the quickest and easiest low carb breakfasts you can make. And even if you are bored with eggs, this recipe is anything but boring. With a filling just like a jalapeño popper, this spicy, creamy omelet takes your breakfast up a notch!

1. In a medium bowl, mash together the cream cheese, 2 tablespoons of the cheddar, and the bacon bits. Stir in the green onions and jalapeño. Set the cream cheese mixture aside.

2. In another medium bowl, whisk together the eggs, heavy cream, sea salt, and black pepper.

3. In a medium skillet, melt the butter over medium heat. Pour in the egg mixture. Cover and cook for 1 to 2 minutes, until mostly cooked through. You can lift with a spatula to get more of the egg underneath if needed, but don't stir or scramble.

4. Drop dollops of the cream cheese mixture onto half of the omelet, distributing as evenly as possible. Use a spatula to fold the omelet over. Sprinkle the remaining 2 tablespoons cheddar cheese on top.

5. Reduce the heat to medium-low. Cover and cook for a couple of minutes, until the cheese melts on top and inside.

TIPS & VARIATIONS • You can taste the cream cheese mixture before adding it to the omelet and adjust the amount of jalapeño based on your heat preference.

• For flavor variations, try chives instead of green onions or Colby Jack cheese instead of cheddar.

1 *ounce (2 tablespoons)* cream cheese, softened at room temperature

4 *tablespoons (1 ounce)* shredded cheddar cheese, divided into 2 tablespoons and 2 tablespoons

2 *tablespoons* cooked bacon bits

1½ *teaspoons* thinly sliced green onions

1½ *teaspoons* finely diced seeded jalapeño pepper (about ⅛ medium)

2 *large* eggs

2 *tablespoons* heavy cream

¼ *teaspoon* sea salt

⅛ *teaspoon* black pepper

1 *tablespoon* butter

MAKES 1 SERVING

SERVING SIZE
1 omelet

PER SERVING
416 calories
35 g fat
3 g total carbs
3 g net carbs
22 g protein

SHEET PAN SAUSAGE BREAKFAST SANDWICHES

Most of the recipes in this book come together quickly, but this one requires a little more prep and time in the kitchen, which I promise is well worth it. In exchange for your hard work, you'll have 12 delicious breakfast sandwiches ready to grab from the freezer and reheat on busy mornings!

1. Preheat the oven to 425°F. Line two 15 × 10-inch jelly-roll pans with parchment paper. Grease well.

2. **Make the pancake layer:** In a large bowl, whisk together all the ingredients.

3. Pour the batter into the lined pans and spread evenly. Bake side by side for 12 to 15 minutes, until firm and golden.

4. Slide the parchment sheets with the pancake layers off the pans and set aside to cool.

5. Leave the oven on at the same temperature. Line both jelly-roll pans with fresh sheets of parchment paper and grease well.

6. **Meanwhile, make the egg layer:** In a large bowl, whisk together the eggs, almond milk, sea salt, and black pepper.

7. Pour the egg mixture into one of the lined pans.

8. Bake for about 15 minutes, or until the egg is firm and cooked through.

9. Slide the parchment sheet with the egg layer off the pan and set aside to cool. Leave the oven on at the same temperature.

recipe continues . . .

PANCAKE LAYER

- 2 *cups (8 ounces)* blanched almond flour
- ¼ *cup* erythritol
- 2 *teaspoons* baking powder
- ¼ *teaspoon* sea salt
- 4 *large* eggs
- ⅔ *cup* unsweetened almond milk
- ¼ *cup* avocado oil
- 1 *teaspoon* vanilla extract
- ½ *teaspoon* real maple extract

EGG LAYER

- 10 *large* eggs
- ½ *cup* unsweetened almond milk
- ½ *teaspoon* sea salt
- ⅛ *teaspoon* black pepper

SAUSAGE LAYER

- 2 *pounds* pork breakfast sausage, no sugar added
- 1 *teaspoon* real maple extract

ASSEMBLY

- 2 *cups (8 ounces)* shredded cheddar cheese

MAKES 12 SERVINGS

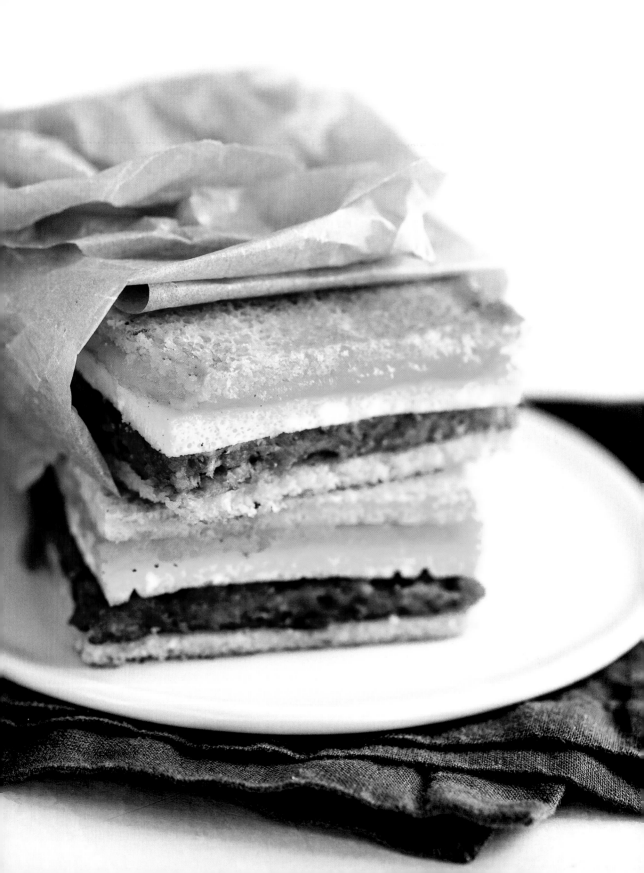

10. **Meanwhile, prepare the sausage layer:** In a medium bowl, mix together the sausage and maple extract. Press the sausage onto the second lined pan in a thin layer, spreading across the entire pan. Press it up the edges of the pan as much as possible, because it will shrink during cooking. (Alternatively, use a slightly larger pan than the other layers, to account for shrinkage of the sausage layer.)

11. Bake for 12 to 16 minutes, until the sausage is cooked through. Drain off the liquid and pat dry with paper towels. Reduce the oven temperature to 350°F.

12. **Assemble the sandwiches:** Carefully slide a large spatula between the parchment paper and one of the pancake layers to release. Repeat with the other pancake layer, egg layer, and sausage layer.

13. Line one of the jelly-roll pans with a fresh sheet of parchment paper. Flip one of the pancake layers onto it, golden side up.

14. Place the sausage layer over the pancake layer, top with the egg layer, and sprinkle cheddar evenly on top. Finally, add the other pancake layer.

15. Return the pan to the oven for about 10 minutes, or until the cheese melts.

16. Let the pan rest for a few minutes, then cut the sheet pan sandwiches into squares. Cut in a grid pattern—3 the short way by 4 the long way, for 12 sandwiches total. Enjoy right away, or cool to room temperature and wrap sandwiches individually in foil, place in a freezer bag, and store in the freezer.

TIPS & VARIATIONS

• If you prefer, you can add cheese twice during the assembly, first on top of the bottom pancake layer and again on top of the egg layer before adding the top pancake layer. This will "glue" the sandwiches together better.

• If you don't like pork, you can also use turkey sausage, or even omit the meat layer. You might want more cheese if you skip the meat.

SERVING SIZE
1 sandwich (5.5 ounces),
$\frac{1}{12}$ of the entire pan

PER SERVING
552 calories
46 g fat
6 g total carbs
3 g net carbs
28 g protein

PROSCIUTTO BAKED EGGS
WITH SPINACH

We usually think of eggs as being cooked on the stove top, but you can bake them, too! The best part is you can make a large batch at once. These prosciutto baked eggs with spinach are ideal for meal prep, or for a crowd. They are versatile enough to serve for friends and family, keto or not!

1. Preheat the oven to 350°F.

2. Place the thawed spinach into a kitchen towel and squeeze well over the sink, getting rid of as much liquid as possible. Set aside.

3. Line 12 cups of a muffin tin with a thin layer of prosciutto, overlapping the prosciutto pieces slightly if necessary. Wrap around the sides first, then patch any holes and the bottom. Set aside.

4. In a large skillet, heat the oil over medium-high heat. Add the minced garlic and sauté for about 30 seconds, until fragrant. Add the spinach and sun-dried tomatoes. Season with the sea salt and black pepper. Sauté for 5 minutes.

5. Divide the spinach mixture evenly among the prosciutto-lined muffin cups. Crack an egg into each muffin cup.

6. Transfer the pan to the oven and bake until the eggs are done to your liking, approximately as follows:

   a. Runny yolks: 13 to 15 minutes

   b. Semi-firm yolks: 16 to 18 minutes

   c. Firm yolks: 18 to 20 minutes

7. Allow the egg muffins to cool in the pan for a few minutes before removing.

1 (12 ounces) bag frozen spinach, thawed and drained

6 ounces prosciutto, very thinly sliced (about 12 large, ultra-thin slices)

1 tablespoon avocado oil

6 cloves garlic, minced

¼ cup finely chopped sun-dried tomatoes

⅛ teaspoon sea salt

Pinch of black pepper

12 large eggs

MAKES 6 SERVINGS

SERVING SIZE
2 egg muffins (5.5 ounces total)

PER SERVING
314 calories
22 g fat
7 g total carbs
5 g net carbs
20 g protein

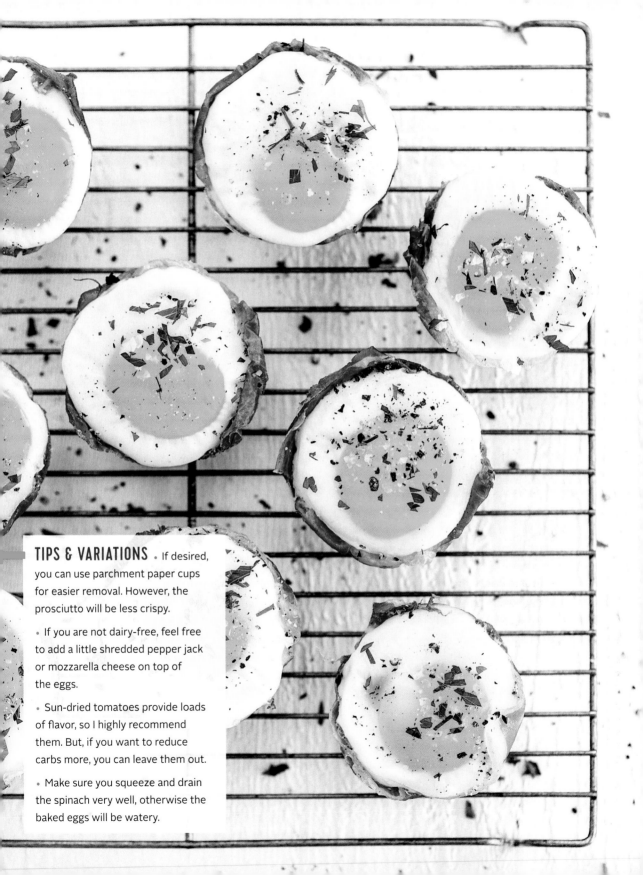

TIPS & VARIATIONS • If desired, you can use parchment paper cups for easier removal. However, the prosciutto will be less crispy.

• If you are not dairy-free, feel free to add a little shredded pepper jack or mozzarella cheese on top of the eggs.

• Sun-dried tomatoes provide loads of flavor, so I highly recommend them. But, if you want to reduce carbs more, you can leave them out.

• Make sure you squeeze and drain the spinach very well, otherwise the baked eggs will be watery.

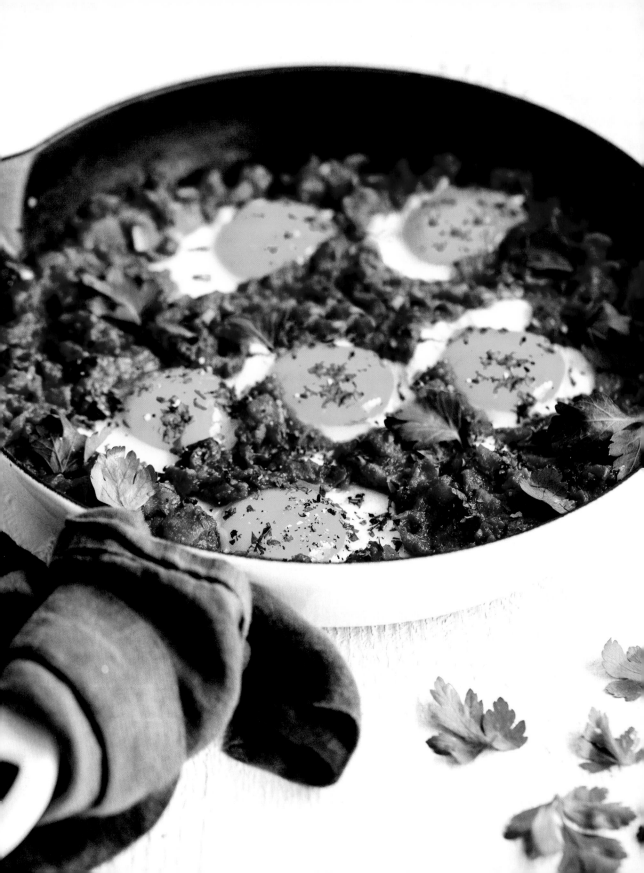

SPICY MEDITERRANEAN SHAKSHUKA

Shakshuka is a Tunisian or Israeli dish consisting of poached eggs in a spicy tomato sauce. This version is one of the easiest ways to make it! It uses common pantry staples and is naturally low carb. Make it as mild or as spicy as you like!

1. In a 12-inch sauté pan, heat the oil over medium-low heat. Add the diced onion and cook for about 10 minutes, until browned. Add the minced garlic and sauté for about 1 minute, until fragrant.

2. Add the diced tomatoes (with juices), tomato sauce, paprika, and cumin and mix. Add the sea salt. Cover and simmer 12 to 15 minutes, until the tomato mixture has thickened and most of the liquid is gone. If needed, cook for a couple of minutes uncovered to reduce.

3. Crack the eggs into the pan so that each egg is surrounded by tomato sauce. If desired, you can create a little well for each egg first. Sprinkle the eggs lightly with more sea salt.

4. Cover and cook for 4 to 6 minutes, until the egg whites are opaque, but the yolks are still runny. If you prefer them more done, continue cooking the eggs to your liking.

5. Sprinkle with parsley to serve.

TIPS & VARIATIONS • This makes a very spicy shakshuka. For a milder version, replace half of the canned diced tomatoes and green chilies with plain canned diced tomatoes.

• If you have a very large (14-inch) pan, you could increase this to 4 servings by using 8 eggs. However, for most typical pan sizes, that many eggs tends to be too crowded.

1 tablespoon avocado oil

½ cup (2 ounces) diced onion

2 cloves garlic, minced

1 (10-ounce) can no-salt-added diced tomatoes with green chilies

½ cup tomato sauce

1 teaspoon paprika

1 teaspoon ground cumin

½ teaspoon sea salt, plus more for taste

6 large eggs

2 tablespoons chopped fresh parsley

MAKES 3 SERVINGS

SERVING SIZE

2 eggs with sauce (7.5 ounces)

PER SERVING

248 calories

15 g fat

10 g total carbs

8 g net carbs

16 g protein

SAVORY BREAKFASTS

55

CRUSTLESS QUICHE LORRAINE

Quiche Lorraine always reminds me of my honeymoon in Paris. The city has a mile-long list of incredible foods to try, but needless to say, many of them aren't low carb. The great news is that quiche Lorraine is one you can easily enjoy on a keto diet by making it crustless. It's so rich and savory, you won't even miss the crust!

1. In a large sauté pan, fry the bacon over medium heat until crispy on both sides. Set aside to drain on paper towels, leaving the bacon grease in the pan.

2. Add the onion to the pan with the bacon grease and sauté over medium heat for about 10 minutes, until translucent and starting to brown. Set aside to cool slightly.

3. Preheat the oven to 350°F. Grease a 9-inch pie pan.

4. In a large bowl, whisk together the eggs, cream, sea salt, cayenne pepper, and chives. Stir in ¾ cup each of the Swiss and Gruyère cheeses.

5. Pour the egg mixture into the prepared pie pan. Sprinkle with the cooked onion. Cut the bacon into small pieces and sprinkle over the eggs. Push the onion and bacon into the eggs. Sprinkle with the remaining ¼ cup each of the Swiss and Gruyère cheeses.

6. Bake for 30 to 40 minutes, until a knife inserted in the center comes out clean.

6 *slices* bacon

½ *cup (~1.5 ounces)* half-moon sliced onion

6 *large* eggs

½ *cup* heavy cream

½ *teaspoon* sea salt

⅛ *teaspoon* cayenne pepper

2 *tablespoons* finely chopped fresh chives

1 *cup (4 ounces)* shredded Swiss cheese, divided into ¾ cup and ¼ cup

1 *cup (4 ounces)* shredded Gruyère cheese, divided into ¾ cup and ¼ cup

MAKES 6 SERVINGS

SERVING SIZE

1 slice (~4 ounces), or ⅙ of entire quiche

PER SERVING

405 calories

33 g fat

3 g total carbs

3 g net carbs

22 g protein

TIPS & VARIATIONS • Feel free to use any cheeses you like. Hard, flavorful cheeses such as Swiss, Gruyère, and cheddar work best.

• You can make the quiche ahead of time. Simply assemble and store in the fridge for up to a few days. Bake right before serving. If you prefer to freeze it, place it in the freezer unbaked and thaw completely before baking.

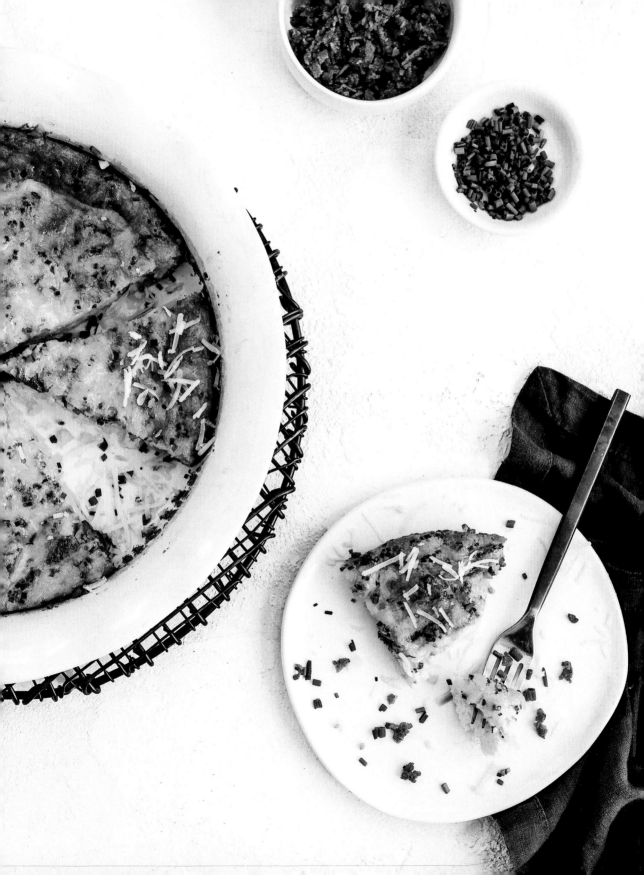

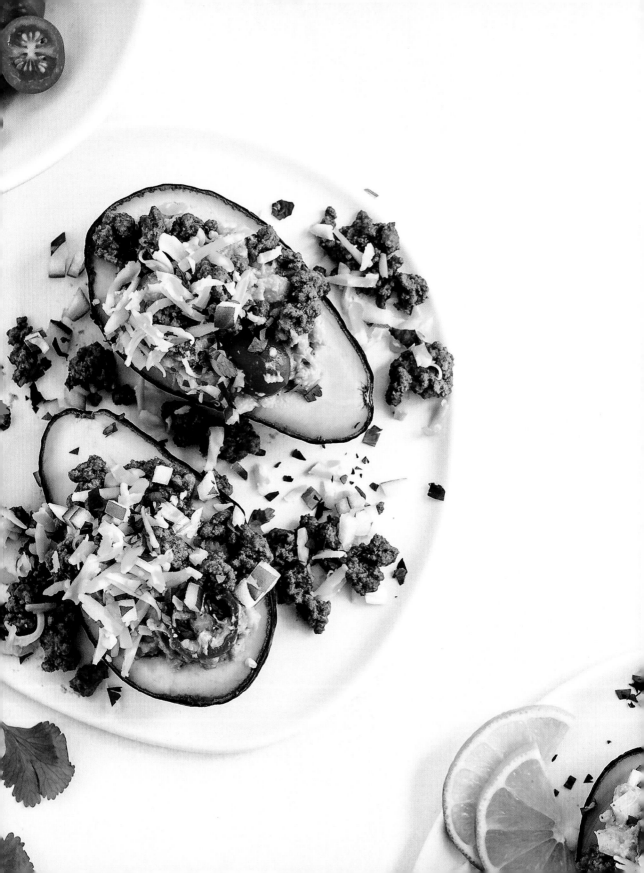

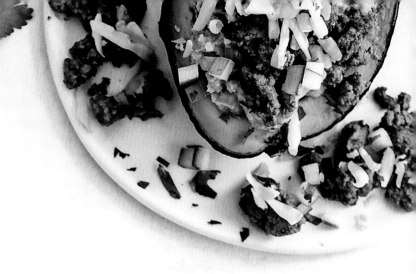

SIMPLE LUNCHES

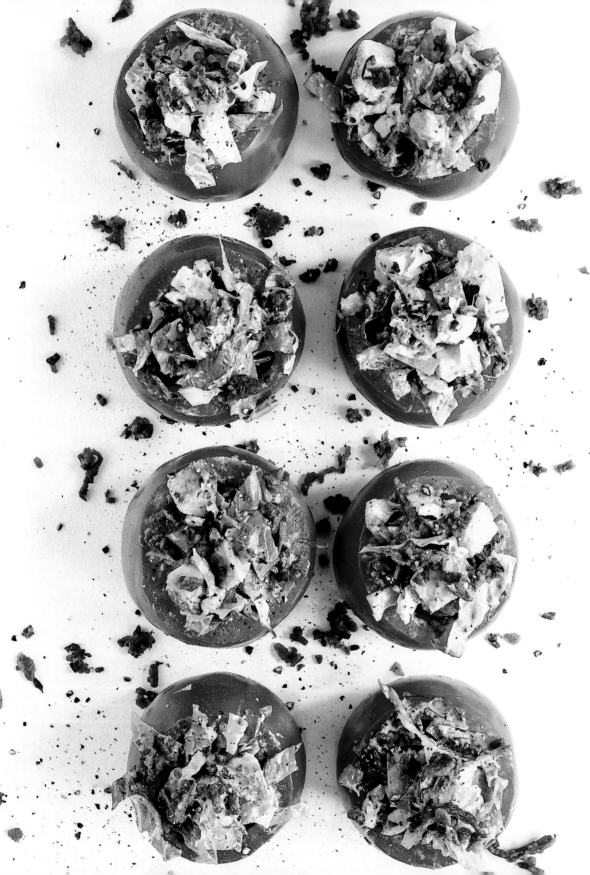

BLTA STUFFED TOMATOES

Who doesn't love a good BLT sandwich? BLTA stuffed tomatoes are a fun twist on a classic. Skip the bread, add some homemade ranch dressing and avocados for good measure, and stuff it all inside the tomatoes instead. So quick and easy for an appetizer or for lunch!

1. Slice the tops off the tomatoes. Cut around the inside, then use a spoon to scoop out and discard the flesh. Flip over and set aside to drain.

2. In a medium bowl, toss together the romaine lettuce, diced avocado, bacon, and ranch dressing.

3. Use paper towels to pat the insides of the tomatoes dry. Stuff the tomatoes with the salad mixture so that they are heaping over the top. Sprinkle lightly with sea salt and black pepper, if desired.

TIPS & VARIATIONS • Buy tomatoes that are wider than they are tall so that they stand up easily. You can also arrange your tomatoes in a muffin tin to stand upright, or cut a thin slice off the bottom of the tomatoes to create a flat, steady base.

• BLTA stuffed tomatoes are best fresh. However, if you want to make these a few hours or a day ahead of time, toss the avocado with a little lime juice before using in the recipe, to reduce browning.

---

8 *medium* tomatoes (~1½ pounds), 2½ to 3 inches in diameter

2 *packed cups* shredded romaine lettuce (~5 ounces)

2 *medium* avocados (6 ounces each), diced

8 *slices* bacon, cooked and chopped

¼ *cup* Ranch Dressing (page 236)

Sea salt and black pepper (optional)

MAKES 4 SERVINGS

SERVING SIZE
2 stuffed tomatoes (~10 ounces total)

PER SERVING
470 calories
41 g fat
19 g total carbs
9 g net carbs
10 g protein

CHICKEN QUESADILLAS

Chicken quesadillas take me back to my college days. They used to be one of my go-to midnight snacks after a night of dancing. Life sure is different now, but my love for quesadillas is the same. Now I make my own keto quesadillas and stock my freezer with them! They make a great lunch that can be heated quickly, or a meal I can grab for my kids at a moment's notice.

1. Toss the chicken pieces with taco seasoning.

2. In a large sauté pan, melt 2 tablespoons of the butter over medium-high heat. Add the chicken and cook for 2 to 3 minutes, until the chicken is browned on the bottom. Flip the chicken and cook for about 2 more minutes, or until cooked through. Remove the chicken from the pan and set aside, leaving behind any remaining butter.

3. Reduce the heat to medium and add the bell pepper to the pan. Cook for a few minutes, stirring occasionally, until soft.

4. In a small bowl, stir together the mayonnaise and salsa. Spread about 1 tablespoon of the mayonnaise/salsa mixture over an entire fathead tortilla, leaving a ½-inch border around the edges. Sprinkle with ¼ cup cheese. Add one-quarter of the chicken and one-quarter of the bell peppers to the tortilla, then top with another ¼ cup cheese. Place a second tortilla on top of the cheese. Repeat this process to create 3 more quesadillas.

5. Wipe down the pan. Add another 1 tablespoon butter to the pan and heat over medium heat until melted.

6. Carefully add 2 of the quesadillas. Cover and cook for a couple of minutes, or until browned on the bottom and cheese starts to melt. Press down onto the top with a spatula before flipping to help the melted cheese stick to the tortilla. Carefully flip and repeat on the other side, until browned on the bottom and the cheese is fully melted.

7. Repeat with the remaining butter and 2 quesadillas.

1 *pound* boneless, skinless chicken breast, cut into 1-inch pieces

½ *teaspoon* Taco Seasoning (page 239)

4 *tablespoons (½ stick)* butter, divided into 2 tablespoons, 1 tablespoon, and 1 tablespoon

½ *cup (2.7 ounces)* 1-inch matchsticks bell pepper

⅓ *cup* 2-Minute Avocado Oil Mayonnaise (page 235)

2 *tablespoons* Pantry Staple Salsa (page 240)

8 *(6-inch)* Pliable Fathead Tortillas (page 201), made with coconut flour or almond flour

2 *cups (8 ounces)* shredded cheddar or pepper jack cheese

MAKES 4 QUESADILLAS

SERVING SIZE
one 6-inch quesadilla

PER SERVING
ALMOND FLOUR VERSION
705 calories
57 g fat
5 g total carbs
4 g net carbs
40 g protein

COCONUT FLOUR VERSION
676 calories
53 g fat
5 g total carbs
4 g net carbs
40 g protein

TIPS & VARIATIONS

• When pan-frying the quesadillas, if the cheese doesn't melt but the tortillas are already browned, you can reduce the heat, cover, and continue cooking in the pan until it melts.

• If you are in a rush, feel free to use store-bought salsa or mayonnaise to save time. Make sure they don't have sugar added. However, the homemade versions are super flavorful!

• Quesadillas store very well. You can make them ahead of time and refrigerate for up to 5 days, or freeze them to have an instant meal anytime.

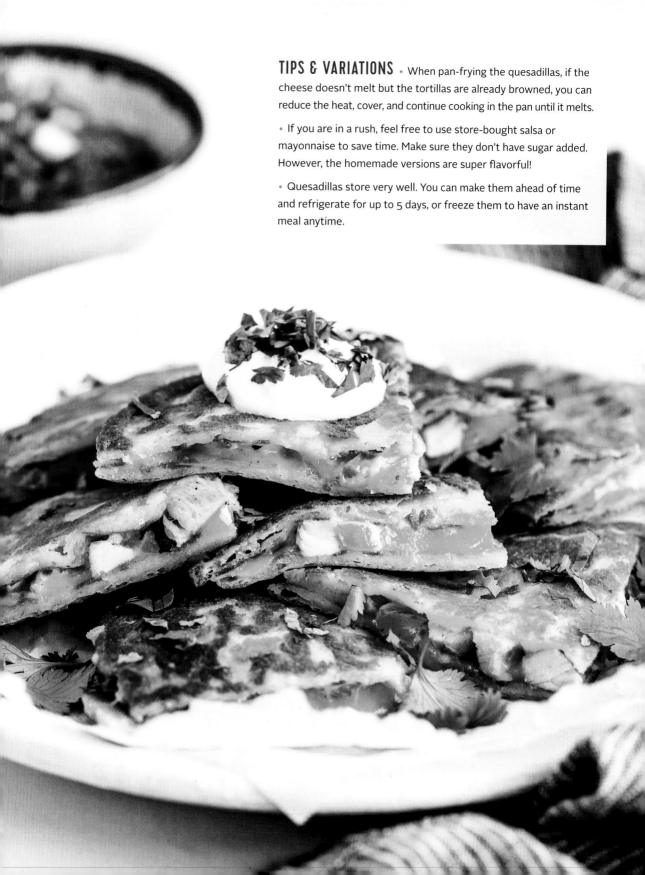

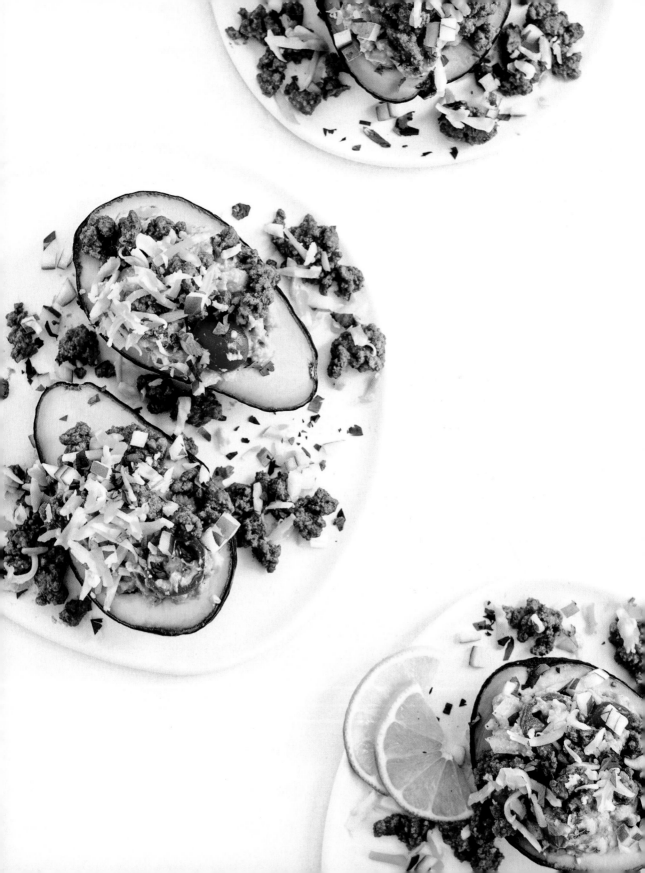

TACO STUFFED AVOCADO

Stuffed avocados are at the top of my list for low carb lunches! They are quick and easy to throw together, especially if you prep the fillings in advance. You can customize them with your favorite fixings, too. And if you love tacos as much as I do, a taco-stuffed avocado is just the thing to satisfy your taco craving without spending the time to make keto tortillas or taco shells (though both are doable!—find them on pages 201 and 193, respectively).

1. In a large skillet, heat the oil over medium-high heat. Add the ground beef and cook, breaking apart with a spatula, 5 to 8 minutes, until cooked through.

2. Add the taco seasoning and ¼ cup water. Sauté for a few minutes, or until the extra liquid is absorbed.

3. Meanwhile, halve the avocados and discard the pits. Scoop most of the avocado flesh out into a large bowl. Set the avocado shells aside.

4. Add the lime juice, sea salt, and black pepper to the scooped-out avocado. Mash together, leaving some pieces. Adjust the lime juice to taste. Add the halved tomatoes and diced onions. Stir together.

5. Stuff the avocado mixture back into the avocado shells. Top with the taco meat, shredded cheese, and cilantro.

> **TIPS & VARIATIONS** • If you are dairy-free, simply omit the cheese.
>
> • You can prepare the taco meat, halved tomatoes, diced onions, and chopped cilantro in advance. However, the avocado should not be prepared in advance, as it will brown quickly.

1 tablespoon avocado oil

½ pound ground beef

1 tablespoon Taco Seasoning (page 239)

2 medium avocados (6 ounces each)

1 teaspoon lime juice, or to taste

¼ teaspoon sea salt

⅛ teaspoon black pepper

½ cup (2.7 ounces) grape tomatoes, halved

¼ cup (1 ounce) diced onions

2 tablespoons (0.5 ounce) shredded Colby Jack cheese

4 teaspoons chopped fresh cilantro

MAKES 4 SERVINGS

SERVING SIZE
½ avocado with filling (5 ounces)

PER SERVING
413 calories
33 g fat
11 g total carbs
4 g net carbs
20 g protein

SIMPLE LUNCHES

CRISPY CHICKEN TENDERS

Even though I love my share of complex flavors and spices, it wasn't always that way. I grew up on simple foods like butter spaghetti and chicken tenders. My palate has come a long way from those days, but I still adore re-creating those childhood comfort foods. Just a few ingredients and simple steps will yield perfectly crispy chicken tenders that are keto-friendly and kid-approved.

½ cup 2-Minute Avocado Oil Mayonnaise (page 235)

2.5 ounces pork rinds, crushed

¼ cup whey protein powder (or collagen protein powder for dairy free)

½ teaspoon garlic powder

½ teaspoon paprika

1½ pounds boneless, skinless chicken breast, cut into 12 strips

MAKES 4 SERVINGS

SERVING SIZE

6 ounces chicken (about 3 chicken strips)

PER SERVING

462 calories

29 g fat

0 g total carbs

0 g net carbs

44 g protein

1. Preheat the oven to 400°F. Line a baking sheet with foil and grease with any fat of your choice.

2. Set up two shallow medium bowls: place the mayonnaise in one and in the other stir together the pork rinds, whey protein powder, garlic powder, and paprika.

3. Toss the chicken strips in the bowl with the mayonnaise. Take a chicken strip from the bowl and remove any excess mayonnaise. Use your other hand to press the chicken strip into the breading mixture and scoop more breading over the top, submerging the chicken strip to coat on all sides. Place on the baking sheet. Repeat with the remaining chicken strips.

4. Bake for 12 to 15 minutes, until just barely cooked through.

5. Turn on the broiler. Place the chicken strips under the broiler for 1 to 2 minutes to crisp up more.

TIPS & VARIATIONS • When dredging the chicken, use both hands: one handling the mayonnaise and the other handling the dry breading. Do not switch hands to avoid getting the dry mixture too wet and clumpy.

• For even crispier chicken tenders, bake them on an ovenproof nonstick wire rack.

• Sprinkle a bit of sea salt over the chicken tenders while they are still hot if you prefer more salt.

• Chicken tenders pair well with Sugar-Free "Honey" Mustard (page 243).

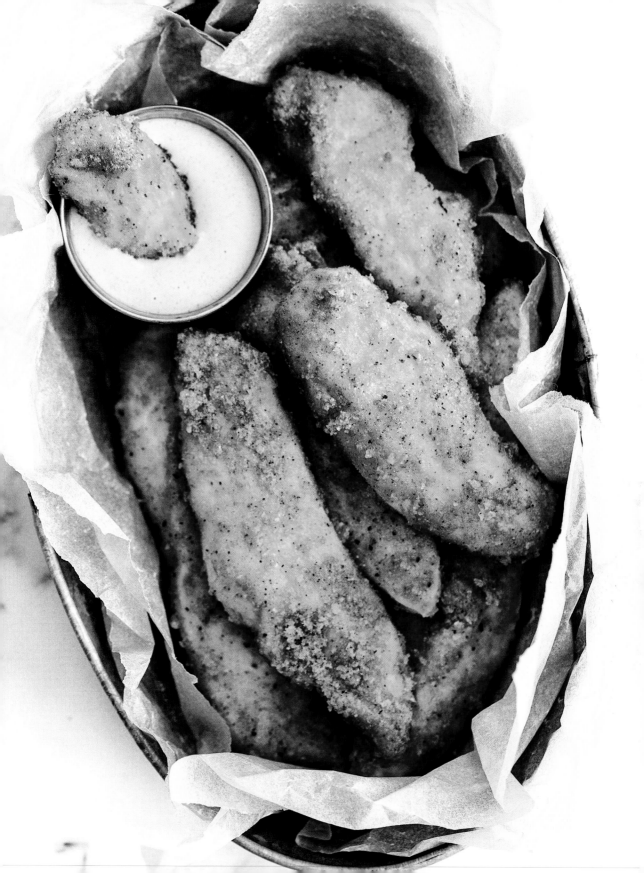

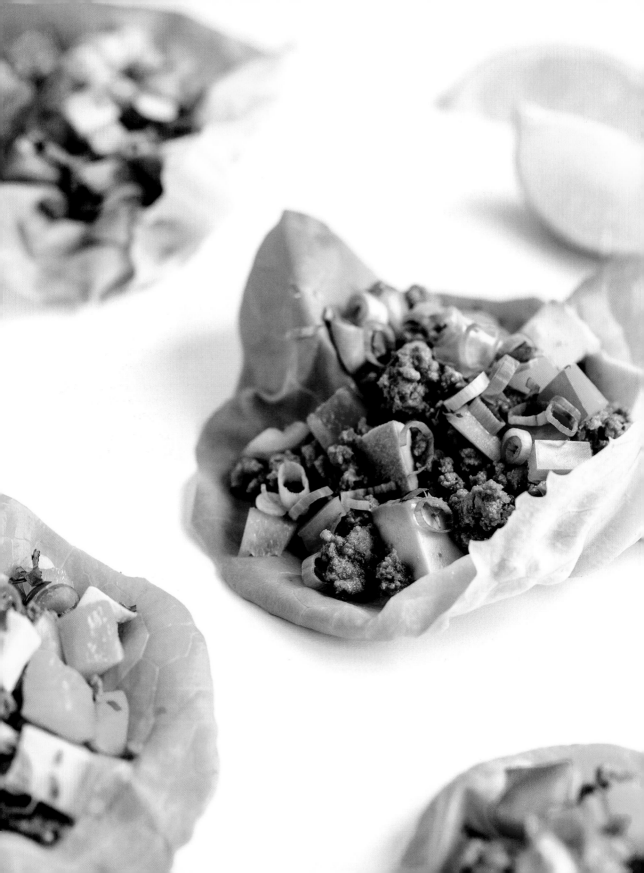

THAI BEEF LETTUCE WRAPS

I love experimenting with international cuisines, but Thai food was something I didn't try until I was in my twenties—and I'm so glad I did! Avoiding sugar and starch can be a challenge in Asian cooking, but you can make just about any dish low carb when it's homemade. Thai beef lettuce wraps are flavorful without the need for added sugar, flour, soy, or dairy. You can even prep the meat in advance, so lunch is ready when you are!

1. In a sauté pan, heat the oil over medium heat. Add the garlic and sauté for about 1 minute, until fragrant. Add the ground beef and season with the sea salt and black pepper. Increase the heat to medium-high and cook, breaking apart with a spatula, about 10 minutes, until browned.

2. Add the coconut aminos, fish sauce, lime juice, and red curry paste. Adjust the curry paste to taste. Cook for 2 to 5 minutes, stirring occasionally, until most of the liquid is evaporated. Add sea salt and black pepper to taste, if needed.

3. Dividing evenly, fill the lettuce leaves with the cooked Thai beef, bell peppers, and diced avocado.

1 tablespoon avocado oil

2 cloves garlic, minced

1 pound ground beef

½ teaspoon sea salt

¼ teaspoon black pepper

3 tablespoons coconut aminos

1 tablespoon fish sauce

1½ tablespoons lime juice

1½ tablespoons red curry paste, or to taste

16 leaves butter lettuce, or any variety of large lettuce leaves

½ cup (2.7 ounces) finely chopped red bell peppers

1 medium (6-ounce) avocado, diced

MAKES 16 LETTUCE WRAPS (4 SERVINGS)

SERVING SIZE

4 small lettuce wraps (½ cup Thai beef, 4 lettuce leaves, 2 tablespoons red pepper, and ¼ avocado; ~6.5 ounces total)

PER SERVING

511 calories
37 g fat
10 g total carbs
6 g net carbs
34 g protein

TIPS & VARIATIONS • Some people prefer their Thai beef to be a little sweet. If you do, add 1 to 2 tablespoons powdered erythritol to taste with the other ingredients in step 3.

• Check the label on the curry paste—make sure you get one without sugar. You can usually find it in the ethnic foods aisle at the grocery store.

• If you don't mind a few extra ingredients, Thai beef lettuce wraps are delicious garnished with green onions, fresh cilantro, and lime wedges.

SIMPLE LUNCHES

LAZY LASAGNA CHICKEN

Baked chicken and lasagna are usually synonymous with dinner, but this lazy lasagna chicken is so quick and easy that you can prep it on the fly for lunch. The prep will only take you 5 to 10 minutes and you can even assemble it in advance. If you take your lunch to work, feel free to bake it ahead—this dish reheats well.

1. Preheat the oven to 375°F.

2. Place the chicken breasts on a sheet pan at least 1 inch apart. Brush both sides of the chicken with melted butter. Season both sides with sea salt and black pepper.

3. In a small bowl, mix together the ricotta and egg, then stir in the Parmesan. Spread evenly over the chicken breasts.

4. Top each piece of chicken with 2 tablespoons marinara sauce, then sprinkle with 2 tablespoons mozzarella.

5. Bake for 23 to 28 minutes, until cooked through. Garnish with fresh basil.

TIPS & VARIATIONS • For a complete meal, serve lasagna chicken over cooked zucchini noodles or spaghetti squash.

• You can make the same recipe with boneless chicken thighs. Just use 8 chicken thighs instead of 4 breasts, and increase the baking time to 28 to 33 minutes.

4 *medium* boneless, skinless chicken breasts (8 ounces each)

2 *tablespoons* butter, melted

½ *teaspoon* sea salt

¼ *teaspoon* black pepper

¼ *cup (2.2 ounces)* ricotta cheese

1 *large* egg

2 *tablespoons (0.5 ounce)* grated Parmesan cheese

½ *cup* marinara sauce, no sugar added

½ *cup (2 ounces)* shredded mozzarella cheese

2 *tablespoons* fresh basil, cut into ribbons

MAKES 4 SERVINGS

SERVING SIZE
1 chicken breast (~8 ounces)

PER SERVING
365 calories
16 g fat
3 g total carbs
3 g net carbs
46 g protein

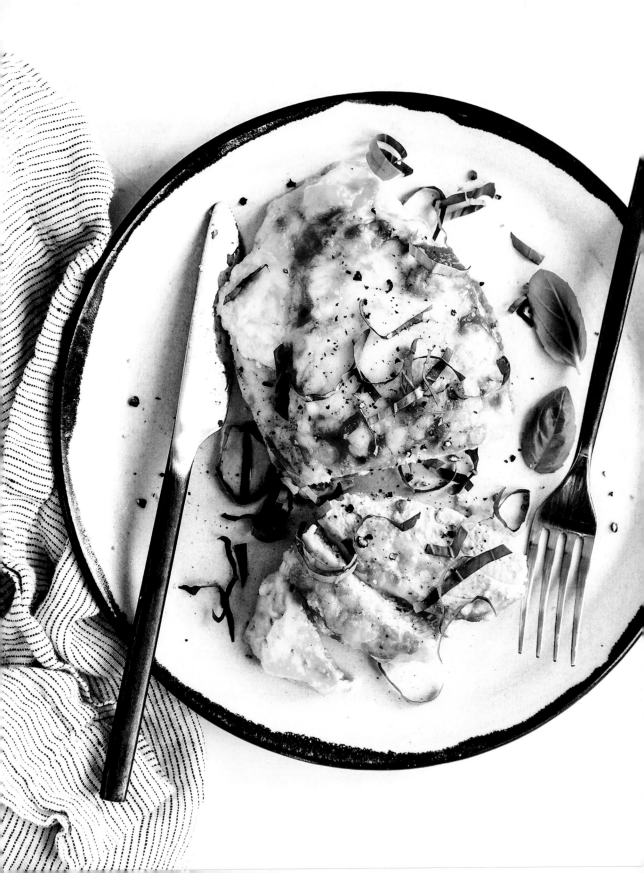

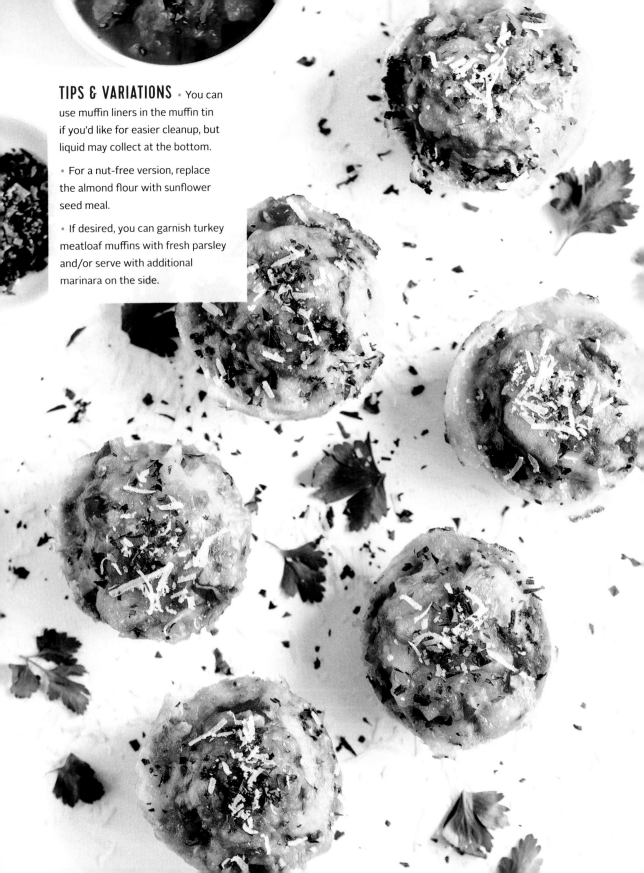

TIPS & VARIATIONS • You can use muffin liners in the muffin tin if you'd like for easier cleanup, but liquid may collect at the bottom.

• For a nut-free version, replace the almond flour with sunflower seed meal.

• If desired, you can garnish turkey meatloaf muffins with fresh parsley and/or serve with additional marinara on the side.

TURKEY MEATLOAF FLORENTINE MUFFINS

I'm a huge fan of preportioned meals you can make ahead of time—especially for lunch! A whole meatloaf is great and all, but meatloaf muffins have their advantages. They are easier to grab and go, plus they cook faster. These turkey meatloaf muffins are stuffed with gooey mozzarella inside, and the spinach keeps the meat ultramoist and tender.

½ *pound* frozen spinach, thawed

2 *pounds* ground turkey

½ *cup (2 ounces)* blanched almond flour

2 *large* eggs

4 *cloves* garlic, minced

2 *teaspoons* sea salt

½ *teaspoon* black pepper

2¼ *cups (9 ounces)* shredded mozzarella cheese, divided into 1½ cups (6 ounces) and ¾ cup (3 ounces)

⅓ *cup* no-sugar-added marinara sauce

MAKES 12 MEATLOAF MUFFINS (6 SERVINGS)

SERVING SIZE
2 muffins (~8 ounces total)

PER SERVING
380 calories
16 g fat
6 g total carbs
4 g net carbs
52 g protein

1. Preheat the oven to 375°F. Lightly grease 12 cups of a muffin tin and place on top of a sheet pan for easier cleanup.

2. Drain the spinach and squeeze it tightly in a kitchen towel to remove as much water as possible.

3. In a large bowl, mix together the spinach, turkey, almond flour, eggs, garlic, sea salt, and black pepper. Mix until just combined, but do not overwork the meat.

4. Fill each muffin cup with 2 tablespoons of the turkey mixture. Create a well with the back of a measuring spoon or your hands. Pack each well with 2 tablespoons mozzarella (1½ cups or 6 ounces total). Top with 2 more tablespoons turkey mixture, lightly pressing down along the sides to seal the filling inside.

5. Spread 1 teaspoon marinara sauce over each meatloaf muffin. Sprinkle each with another 1 tablespoon mozzarella (¾ cup or 3 ounces total).

6. Bake for 20 to 25 minutes, until the internal temperature reaches at least 160°F. Let rest for 5 minutes before serving (temperature will rise another 5 degrees while resting).

SUN-DRIED TOMATO AND ARUGULA AVOCADO TOAST

I fell in love with avocado toast the first time I tried it! You may be wondering what it's doing in a keto cookbook, but why not? You can totally make it using low carb bread. The combination of avocado, arugula, garlic, and sun-dried tomatoes makes an incredibly flavorful topping, which also happens to be dairy-free and meatless.

1. Toast the bread to desired doneness.

2. Meanwhile, in a bowl, mash together the avocado, garlic, sea salt, and black pepper. Adjust the sea salt and black pepper to taste, if desired.

3. Spread the avocado mash over the toast. Top with arugula and sun-dried tomatoes. Drizzle with olive oil.

TIPS & VARIATIONS • If desired, you can liven this up with a coarse-grain sea salt, freshly cracked black pepper, and/or a drizzle of lemon juice on top.

• A fried egg also makes a delicious addition to avocado toast.

• For the dairy-free option, make the dairy-free version of the Easy All-Purpose Bread used in this recipe.

4 *slices (¾ inch thick)* Easy All-Purpose Bread (page 197), about one-third of the recipe

2 *medium* avocados (6 ounces each)

1 *clove* garlic, minced

½ *teaspoon* sea salt, or to taste

¼ *teaspoon* black pepper, or to taste

1 *packed cup (1 ounce)* arugula

8 *teaspoons* chopped sun-dried tomatoes, packed in oil

2 *tablespoons* extra virgin olive oil

MAKES 4 SERVINGS

SERVING SIZE
1 piece of toast (4 to 5 ounces)

PER SERVING
453 calories
38 g fat
23 g total carbs
9 g net carbs
10 g protein

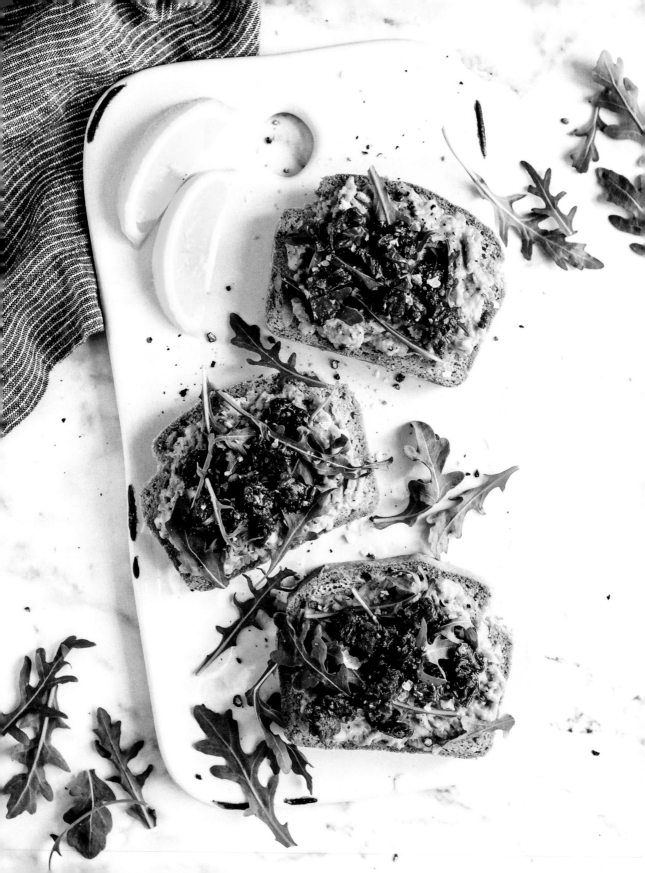

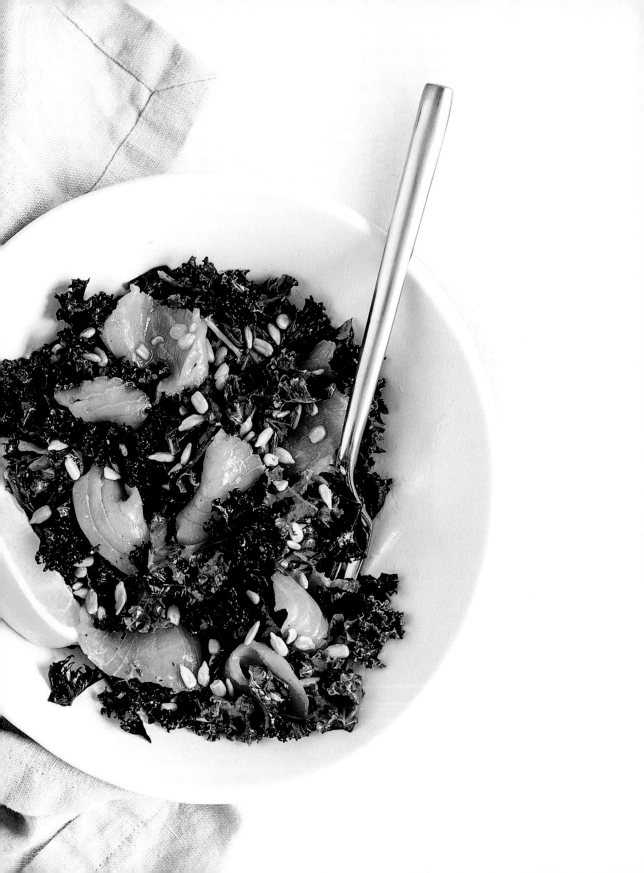

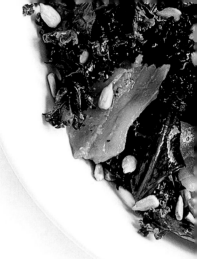

HEARTY SOUPS & SALADS

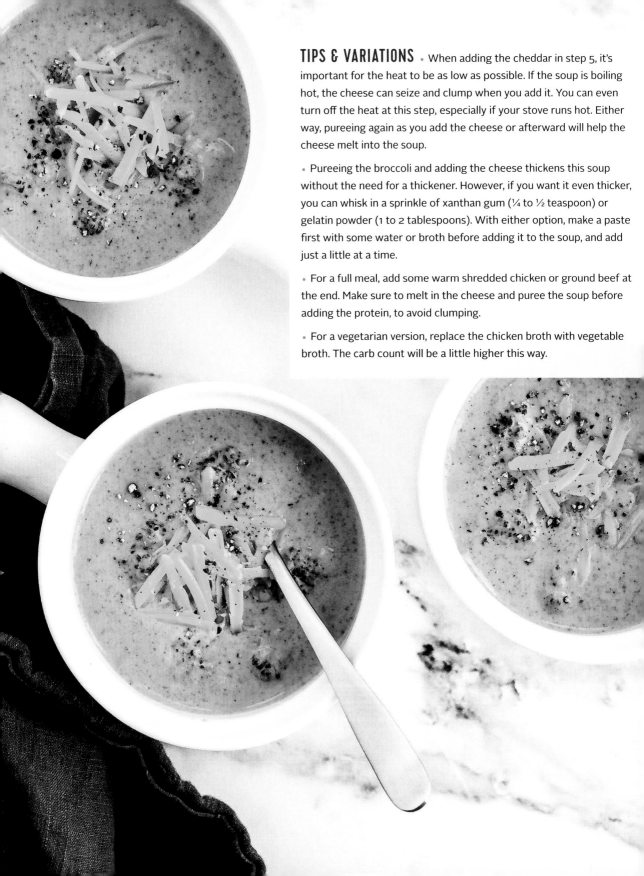

TIPS & VARIATIONS • When adding the cheddar in step 5, it's important for the heat to be as low as possible. If the soup is boiling hot, the cheese can seize and clump when you add it. You can even turn off the heat at this step, especially if your stove runs hot. Either way, pureeing again as you add the cheese or afterward will help the cheese melt into the soup.

• Pureeing the broccoli and adding the cheese thickens this soup without the need for a thickener. However, if you want it even thicker, you can whisk in a sprinkle of xanthan gum (¼ to ½ teaspoon) or gelatin powder (1 to 2 tablespoons). With either option, make a paste first with some water or broth before adding it to the soup, and add just a little at a time.

• For a full meal, add some warm shredded chicken or ground beef at the end. Make sure to melt in the cheese and puree the soup before adding the protein, to avoid clumping.

• For a vegetarian version, replace the chicken broth with vegetable broth. The carb count will be a little higher this way.

5-INGREDIENT BROCCOLI CHEESE SOUP

Broccoli cheese soup was one of the first Wholesome Yum recipes that became really popular among readers. This recipe has gone through several revisions since then, but it's still a reader favorite and a family staple at our house. It's smooth, creamy, *super* cheesy, and so comforting on a chilly day. You won't believe you need just 5 ingredients to make it!

4   *cloves* garlic, minced

3½ *cups* chicken broth

1   *cup* heavy cream

4   *cups (8 ounces)* broccoli florets

3   *cups (12 ounces)* shredded cheddar cheese

MAKES 6 SERVINGS*

1. In a large pot, cook the garlic over medium heat for 1 minute, until fragrant. (You can add a little butter to sauté it in if you'd like.)

2. Add the chicken broth, cream, and broccoli. Increase the heat to bring to a boil, then reduce the heat and simmer for 10 to 20 minutes, until the broccoli is tender.

3. Use a slotted spoon to remove about one-third of the broccoli pieces and set aside. (This step is optional, if you want some broccoli florets in your soup at the end. If you want all of the soup pureed, you can leave them in.)

4. Use an immersion blender to puree the mixture, or transfer to a regular blender in batches if you don't have an immersion blender.

5. Reduce the heat to low. Add the cheddar ½ cup at a time, stirring constantly, and continue to stir until melted. Puree again until smooth.

6. Remove from the heat. Return the reserved broccoli florets to the soup.

SERVING SIZE

1 cup
*Number of servings will vary slightly depending on how much of the broccoli you puree.

PER SERVING

394 calories
33 g fat
7 g total carbs
6 g net carbs
17 g protein

HEARTY SOUPS & SALADS

CAULIFLOWER "POTATO" SALAD

You're probably wondering how it's possible to create a keto potato salad. We do it with the best potato replacement: cauliflower! Even if you're skeptical about cauliflower, I encourage you to give this a try, because it has all the flavors of a potato salad. And the flavors only improve over time, making this a great make-ahead salad.

1. **Stovetop method:** Bring a pot of water to a boil with the salt. Add the cauliflower and simmer until very tender, about 5 minutes. Drain well and allow to cool.

   Microwave method: Place the cauliflower florets in a large bowl with 2 tablespoons water, and cover with plastic wrap without touching the cauliflower. Microwave on high for 10 minutes, stirring halfway through. Drain well.

2. Meanwhile, in a large bowl, whisk together the mayonnaise, vinegar, mustard, garlic powder, paprika, sea salt, and black pepper until smooth.

3. Add the cauliflower, onion, celery, and eggs to the dressing and toss to coat. Garnish with the chives and additional paprika, if desired.

TIPS & VARIATIONS · For a consistency similar to potato salad, make sure the cauliflower florets are cut very small and cooked until very soft.

• Crumbled bacon or diced ham make great additions!

1 *tablespoon* salt

1 *head* cauliflower, cut into small florets (~4 cups or 2 pounds florets)

⅔ *cup* 2-Minute Avocado Oil Mayonnaise (page 235)

1 *tablespoon* apple cider vinegar

1 *tablespoon* Dijon mustard

½ *teaspoon* garlic powder

½ *teaspoon* paprika, plus more for garnish (optional)

½ *teaspoon* sea salt

¼ *teaspoon* black pepper

⅓ *cup (3 ounces)* finely diced onion

⅓ *cup (3 ounces)* finely diced celery

2 *large* eggs, hard-boiled and chopped

1 *tablespoon* chopped chives (optional)

MAKES 5 CUPS (5 SERVINGS)

SERVING SIZE
1 cup (5.7 ounces)

PER SERVING
250 calories
21 g fat
11 g total carbs
6 g net carbs
6 g protein

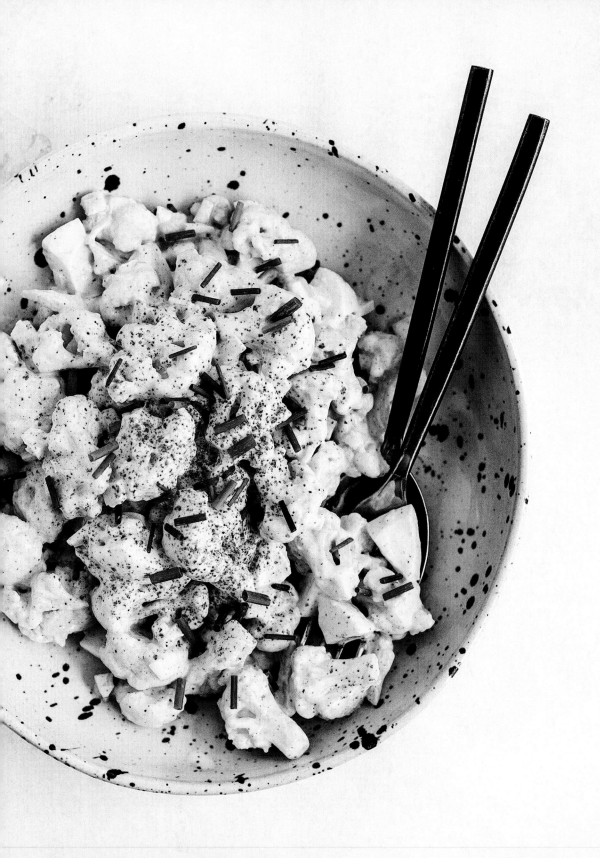

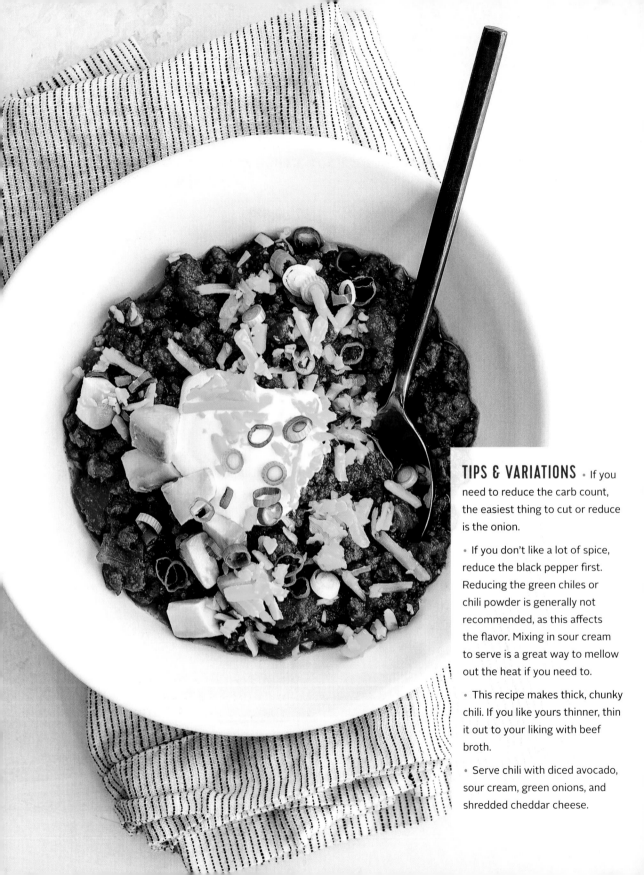

TIPS & VARIATIONS • If you need to reduce the carb count, the easiest thing to cut or reduce is the onion.

• If you don't like a lot of spice, reduce the black pepper first. Reducing the green chiles or chili powder is generally not recommended, as this affects the flavor. Mixing in sour cream to serve is a great way to mellow out the heat if you need to.

• This recipe makes thick, chunky chili. If you like yours thinner, thin it out to your liking with beef broth.

• Serve chili with diced avocado, sour cream, green onions, and shredded cheddar cheese.

CLASSIC HEARTY BEEF CHILI

Chili may seem like a naturally low carb food, but beans are actually quite high in carbs. Fortunately, it's easy to make a keto-friendly chili by leaving them out. With the right combination of spices, you'll get a hearty, chunky chili with all the same flavors you love.

1 tablespoon olive oil

½ large onion (5.5 ounces), chopped

8 cloves garlic, minced

2½ pounds ground beef

2 (14.5-ounce) cans diced tomatoes, with liquid

1 (6-ounce) can tomato paste

1 (4-ounce) can green chiles, with liquid

¼ cup chili powder

2 tablespoons ground cumin

1 tablespoon dried oregano

2 teaspoons sea salt

1 teaspoon black pepper

1 medium bay leaf (optional)

MAKES 10 CUPS
(10 SERVINGS)

SERVING SIZE
1 cup (~7.5 ounces)

PER SERVING
427 calories
27 g fat
10 g total carbs
8 g net carbs
33 g protein

SLOW COOKER METHOD:

1. In a large skillet, heat the oil over medium-high heat. Add the onion and cook for 5 to 7 minutes, until translucent, or longer if you like it caramelized. Add the garlic and cook for 1 minute or less, until fragrant.

2. Add the ground beef and cook for 8 to 10 minutes, breaking apart with a spatula, until browned.

3. Transfer the ground beef mixture to a slow cooker. Add the remaining ingredients, except the bay leaf, and stir until combined. If desired, place the bay leaf in the middle and push down slightly.

4. Cook on low for 6 to 8 hours or on high for 3 to 4 hours. Remove the bay leaf before serving.

STOVETOP METHOD:

1. In a soup pot or Dutch oven, heat the oil over medium-high heat. Add the onion and cook for 5 to 7 minutes, until translucent, or longer if you like it caramelized. Add the garlic and cook for 1 minute or less, until fragrant.

2. Add the ground beef and cook for 8 to 10 minutes, breaking apart with a spatula, until browned.

3. Add the remaining ingredients, except the bay leaf, and stir until combined. If desired, place the bay leaf in the middle and push down slightly.

4. Reduce heat to low. Cover and cook for 1 hour, or until the flavors reach the desired intensity. Remove the bay leaf before serving.

SAUSAGE ZOODLE SOUP

A comforting bowl of soup is perfect for warming up on cold days! Sausage zoodle soup needs just a few simple ingredients, and the zucchini noodles will satisfy a craving for pasta. It's also super filling, without many carbs or calories.

1. In a large soup pot, heat the oil over medium heat. Add the garlic and cook for about 1 minute, until fragrant.

2. Add the sausage, increase the heat to medium-high, and cook for about 10 minutes, stirring occasionally and breaking apart into small pieces, until browned.

3. Add the seasoning, regular broth, and bone broth, and simmer for 10 minutes.

4. Add the zucchini. Bring to a simmer again, then simmer for about 2 minutes, until the zucchini is soft. (Don't overcook or the zoodles will be mushy.)

1 *tablespoon* olive oil

4 *cloves* garlic, minced

1 *pound* pork sausage (no sugar added)

½ *tablespoon* Italian seasoning

3 *cups* regular beef broth

3 *cups* beef bone broth

2 *medium* zucchini (6 ounces each), spiralized

MAKES 8 CUPS (8 SERVINGS)

SERVING SIZE
1 cup (~9 ounces)

PER SERVING
216 calories
17 g fat
2 g total carbs
2 g net carbs
12 g protein

TIPS & VARIATIONS • For the best flavor and health benefits, use a 50/50 combination of beef bone broth and regular beef broth (3 cups each). For convenience, you can use just one or the other.

• Browning the pork sausage to a darker brown over higher heat will create more flavor. The best temperature might be medium-high or high, depending on your stove.

• Before adding the spiralized zucchini to the soup, use kitchen shears to cut them into manageable noodle lengths for eating.

• Feel free to mix it up by adding other veggies. Aromatics, such as onions, should be cooked before browning the meat. Harder veggies that take longer to cook, such as radishes, can go in together with the broth. Veggies that soften or wilt quickly, such as spinach, can be added in the last few minutes with the zoodles.

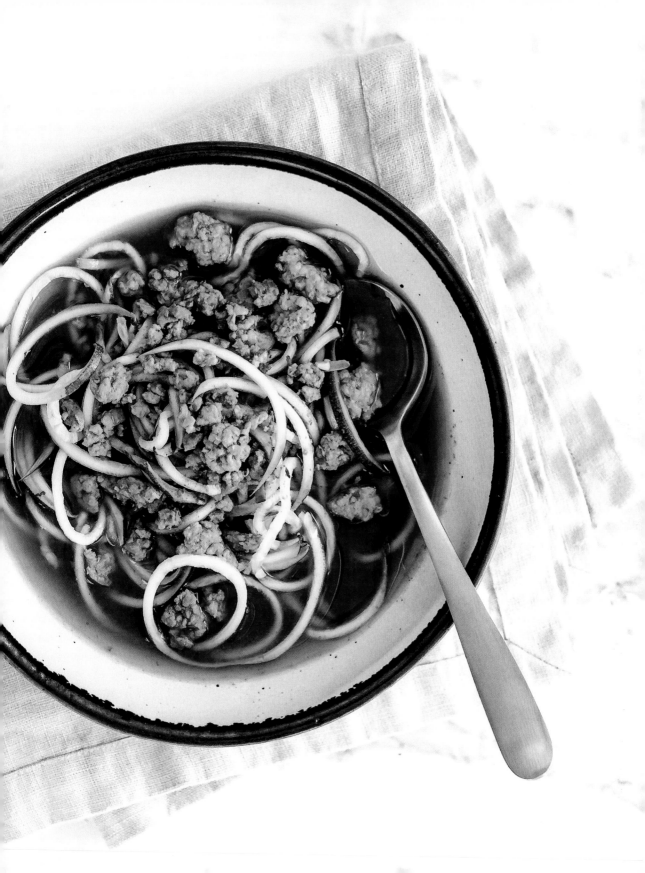

TIPS & VARIATIONS • Make sure the oil and pan are very hot before adding the steak. This will ensure it gets a nicely browned exterior for the best flavor.

• Steak cook time will depend on your pan, your stove, and how thick the steak is sliced. For best results, slice against the grain as thinly as possible, ⅛ to ¼ inch thick. It may help to place the steak in the freezer first to help with making the slices thinner.

• Feel free to add other Southwestern flavors, such as a handful of chopped cilantro, diced red onion, or a squeeze of lime. Avoid higher-carb add-ins such as beans or corn.

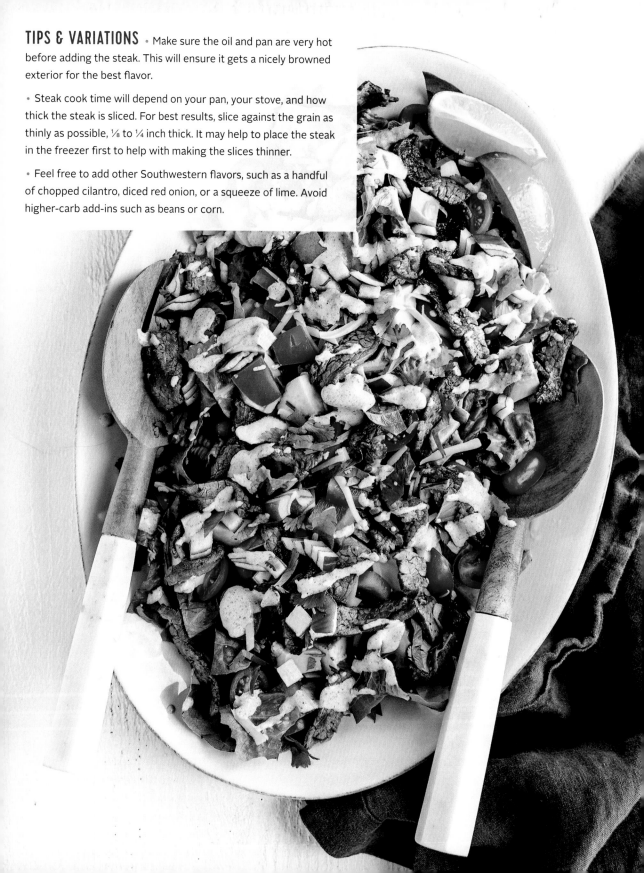

SOUTHWESTERN RANCH STEAK SALAD

On busy weeknights, it's a pretty regular occurrence for me to throw together a big salad and call it a day. You have your protein, greens, a variety of veggies, sharp cheese, and in this case, zesty Southwestern ranch dressing—loads of flavor without too much effort. Even though we skip the usual beans and corn, this salad still carries all the same flavors you'd expect from Southwestern cuisine.

1. **Prepare the steak:** In a large bowl, season the steak with sea salt and black pepper. Drizzle with 1 tablespoon of the oil and stir to coat. Set aside to rest while preparing the remaining ingredients.

2. **Make the Southwestern ranch dressing:** In a bowl, whisk together the ranch dressing, chili powder, and cumin. Add more chili powder to taste if you like it spicy. Set aside.

3. **Prepare the salad:** In a large bowl, place the lettuce, bell pepper, tomatoes, avocado, and cheddar. Set aside.

4. In a large skillet, heat the remaining 1 tablespoon oil over high heat. Working in batches if needed, add the steak in a single layer. Cook for 2 to 4 minutes, without moving, until browned on the bottom. Flip and repeat on the other side. If the steak is not cooked through, stir-fry as needed until it is. Repeat with the remaining beef.

5. Toss the salad with the dressing. Serve slices of steak on top of each portion of salad.

STEAK

- 1 *pound* flank steak, very thinly sliced against the grain
- 1 *teaspoon* sea salt
- ¼ *teaspoon* black pepper
- 2 *tablespoons* avocado oil, divided into 1 tablespoon and 1 tablespoon

SOUTHWESTERN RANCH DRESSING

- ¼ *cup* Ranch Dressing (page 236)
- ½ *teaspoon* chili powder, or to taste
- ½ *teaspoon* ground cumin

SALAD

- 6 *cups (16 ounces)* chopped romaine lettuce
- 1 *large (7-ounce)* bell pepper, chopped
- 1½ *cups (8 ounces)* grape tomatoes, halved
- 1 *medium (6-ounce)* avocado, diced
- ½ *cup (2 ounces)* shredded cheddar cheese

MAKES 12 CUPS
(6 SERVINGS)

SERVING SIZE
2 cups salad + 2.5 ounces meat
(9 ounces total)

PER SERVING
311 calories
22 g fat
8 g total carbs
4 g net carbs
20 g protein

HEARTY SOUPS & SALADS

SMOKED SALMON KALE SALAD

Many people steer clear of kale, worrying that it can be bitter, but it doesn't have to be! Kale can be delicious if you make it the right way. The key is to massage the greens in oil and lemon juice to soften them, which makes the kale easier to chew while getting rid of the bitterness. Give it a try and you might be pleasantly surprised!

1. In a large bowl, whisk together the olive oil, lemon juice, garlic powder, sea salt, and black pepper.

2. Add the chopped kale. Use your hands to massage the kale with the dressing mixture. Grab a bunch, squeeze with the dressing, release, and repeat. Do this for a couple of minutes, until the kale starts to soften.

3. Add the sunflower seeds and smoked salmon. Toss together.

TIPS & VARIATIONS • Unlike most other green salads, massaged kale salad can be prepared a few hours in advance of serving, or even overnight. However, it tastes best cold, so refrigerate it. The seeds are best added right before eating.

• Replace sunflower seeds with walnuts, pecans, or sliced almonds if you prefer.

• If you are not dairy-free, crumbled goat cheese makes a nice addition.

• The serving size of 1 cup is an appetizer portion. If you are having this as an entrée, I recommend doubling the serving size (and the recipe, if you want to make 4 servings).

¼ cup **extra virgin olive oil**

1 tablespoon **lemon juice**

½ teaspoon **garlic powder**

½ teaspoon **sea salt**

¼ teaspoon **black pepper**

6 ounces **chopped and deribbed kale (from 8 to 10 ounces untrimmed)**

¼ cup **salted roasted sunflower seeds**

8 ounces **smoked salmon, cut into pieces**

MAKES 4 APPETIZER SERVINGS

SERVING SIZE
1 packed cup (~4.5 ounces)

PER SERVING
257 calories
20 g fat
6 g total carbs
6 g net carbs
14 g protein

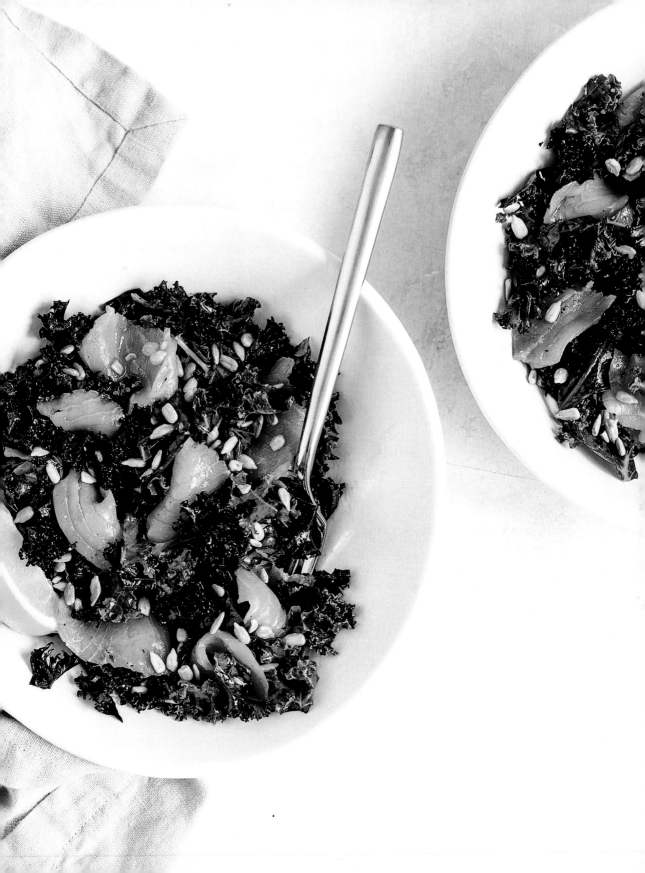

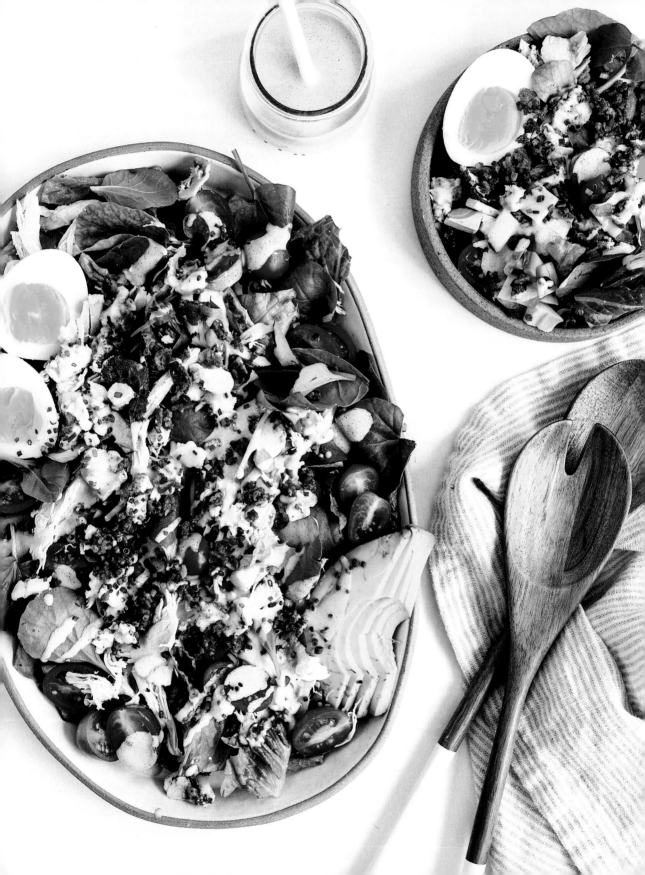

HONEY-MUSTARD CHICKEN COBB SALAD

If I had to pick one salad that is my absolute favorite, it's a Cobb salad, hands down! Not only is it packed with flavor, but this salad is naturally brimming with ingredients ideal for the keto lifestyle. Bacon? Check. Avocado? Check. Greens and low carb veggies? Check. And the sugar-free honey-mustard dressing takes it over the top!

In a large bowl, combine all the ingredients except the honey-mustard dressing, sea salt, and black pepper. Add the honey-mustard dressing and toss to combine. Season to taste with the sea salt and black pepper.

TIPS & VARIATIONS
· For a dairy-free option, simply omit the cheese.

· If you like a little crunch, add a handful of walnuts or sunflower seeds.

· If the honey-mustard dressing is too thick and difficult to mix in, you can thin it out with 2 teaspoons olive oil and 1 teaspoon apple cider vinegar.

· To save time making this recipe, use store-bought bacon bits and rotisserie chicken.

5 cups (13 ounces) chopped romaine lettuce

5 cups (7.5 ounces) chopped watercress

8 slices bacon, cooked and cut into small pieces or crumbled

12 ounces boneless, skinless chicken breast, cooked and cut into cubes or shredded

2 cups (10.6 ounces) grape tomatoes, halved

2 medium avocados (6 ounces each)

4 large eggs, hard-boiled and diced or sliced

½ cup (2 ounces) Roquefort cheese, crumbled

2 tablespoons finely chopped chives

½ cup Sugar-Free "Honey" Mustard (page 243)

Sea salt and black pepper

MAKES 16 CUPS (8 SERVINGS)

SERVING SIZE
2 cups (~10 ounces)

PER SERVING
366 calories
28 g fat
9 g total carbs
5 g net carbs
19 g protein

HEARTY SOUPS & SALADS

SPAGHETTI SQUASH RAMEN SOUP

Ramen soup isn't just for college students! I was never a fan of the packaged stuff anyway, and it turns out that making your own is much more fun. Of course, my keto version has no rice noodles—I use spaghetti squash in their place, for fewer carbs and more fiber and nutrients. You're going to love the umami flavors in this keto-fied ramen soup!

1. Preheat the oven to 425°F. Line a baking sheet with foil and grease lightly.

2. **Prepare the spaghetti squash:** Use a sharp chef's knife to slice the spaghetti squash in half. To make it easier, use the knife to score where you'll be cutting first, then slice. Cut crosswise to yield longer noodles, or lengthwise for shorter ones. Scoop out the seeds.

3. Drizzle the inside of the halves with the avocado oil. Sprinkle lightly with sea salt.

4. Place the spaghetti squash halves on the lined baking sheet cut side down. Roast for 25 to 35 minutes, until the skin pierces easily with a knife. The knife should be able to go in pretty deep with very slight resistance.

5. Remove from the oven and let the squash rest on the pan (cut side down, without moving) for 10 minutes. Then use a fork to release the strands inside the shells and set aside.

6. **Meanwhile, make the soup:** In a large soup pot, heat the oil over medium heat. Add the garlic and ginger and sauté for about 1 minute, until fragrant.

7. Add the shiitake mushrooms and sauté for about 5 minutes, or until the mushrooms are soft.

8. Add the chicken broth, coconut aminos, and fish sauce (if using). Add salt to taste (start with 1 teaspoon salt and add more if needed, but I recommend 1½ teaspoons). Bring to a boil, then reduce the heat and simmer for 10 minutes.

SPAGHETTI SQUASH

1 *medium (2-pound)* **spaghetti squash**

2 *tablespoons* **avocado oil**

Sea salt

SOUP

1 *tablespoon* **avocado oil**

4 *cloves* **garlic, minced**

1 *tablespoon* **minced fresh ginger**

2 *cups (5 ounces)* **shiitake mushrooms, sliced**

8 *cups* **chicken broth**

⅓ *cup* **coconut aminos**

1 *tablespoon* **fish sauce (optional)**

1½ *teaspoons* **sea salt, or to taste**

GARNISHES

¼ *cup (0.9 ounce)* **chopped green onions**

4 *large* **eggs, soft-boiled, peeled, and cut in half**

MAKES 8 CUPS (4 SERVINGS)

SERVING SIZE
2 cups soup (16 ounces) with 1 soft-boiled egg

PER SERVING
238 calories
16 g fat
10 g total carbs
10 g net carbs
10 g protein

9. Add the spaghetti squash noodles to the pot and simmer for 10 to 15 minutes, until hot and flavors develop to your liking.

10. Pour into bowls. Garnish with the green onions and soft-boiled eggs.

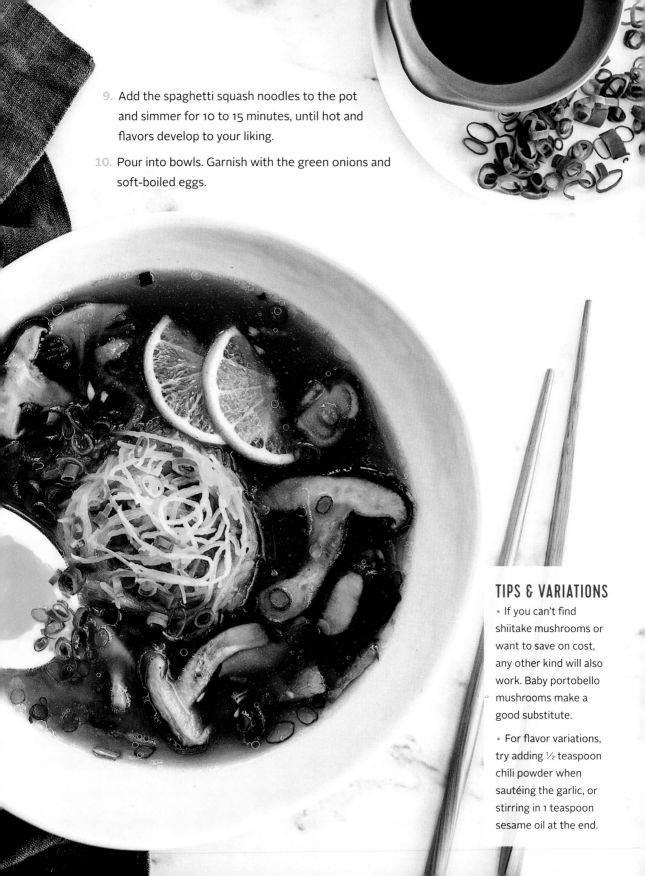

TIPS & VARIATIONS

• If you can't find shiitake mushrooms or want to save on cost, any other kind will also work. Baby portobello mushrooms make a good substitute.

• For flavor variations, try adding ½ teaspoon chili powder when sautéing the garlic, or stirring in 1 teaspoon sesame oil at the end.

GREEK HORIATIKI ZUCCHINI SALAD

I spent time in college working in a Greek restaurant, and one of the things I learned is that traditional Greek salads actually aren't made with any leafy greens. I re-created my favorite *horiatiki* salad from that restaurant in this recipe, but threw in some zucchini to add more volume with minimal carbs. It's simple, it's delicious, and it screams summertime!

1. In a large bowl, combine all the ingredients except the dressing.

2. Pour the dressing over the salad and toss to coat.

TIPS & VARIATIONS • Salad can get watery upon standing. For best results, stir in the dressing right before serving.

• If you want to cut carbs a bit more, omit or reduce the onions.

• For a dairy-free version, simply omit the cheese.

3 cups (16 ounces) grape tomatoes, halved

2 cups (10 ounces) diced cucumbers

1½ cups (7 ounces) diced zucchini

½ cup (2.5 ounces) Kalamata olives

½ cup (2 ounces) red onion quarter-moons

½ cup (2.5 ounces) crumbled feta cheese

1 recipe Basic Greek Vinaigrette (page 251)

MAKES 8 SERVINGS

SERVING SIZE
1 cup (~4 ounces)

PER SERVING
139 calories
12 g fat
5 g total carbs
4 g net carbs
2 g protein

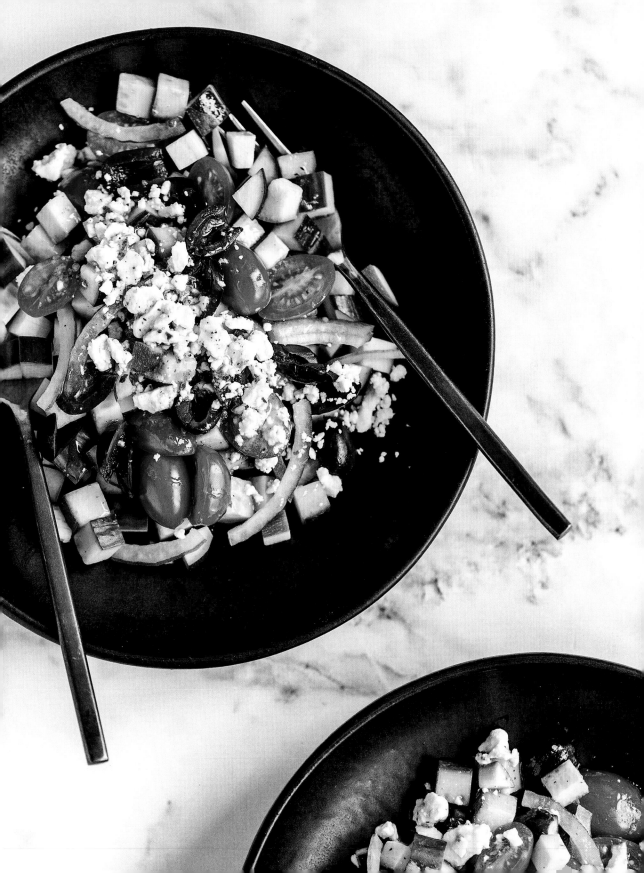

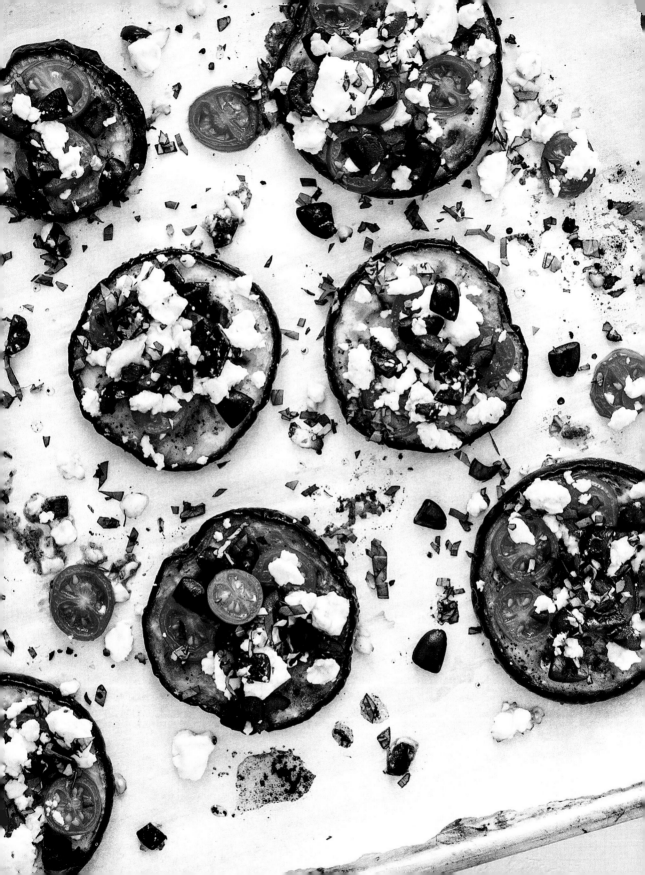

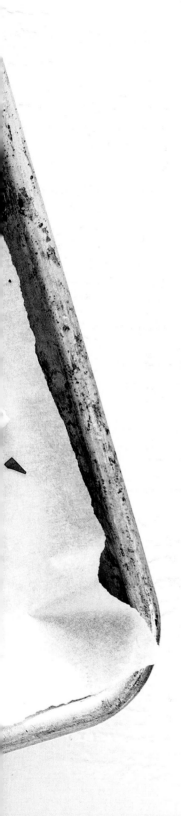

ONE-PAN MEALS

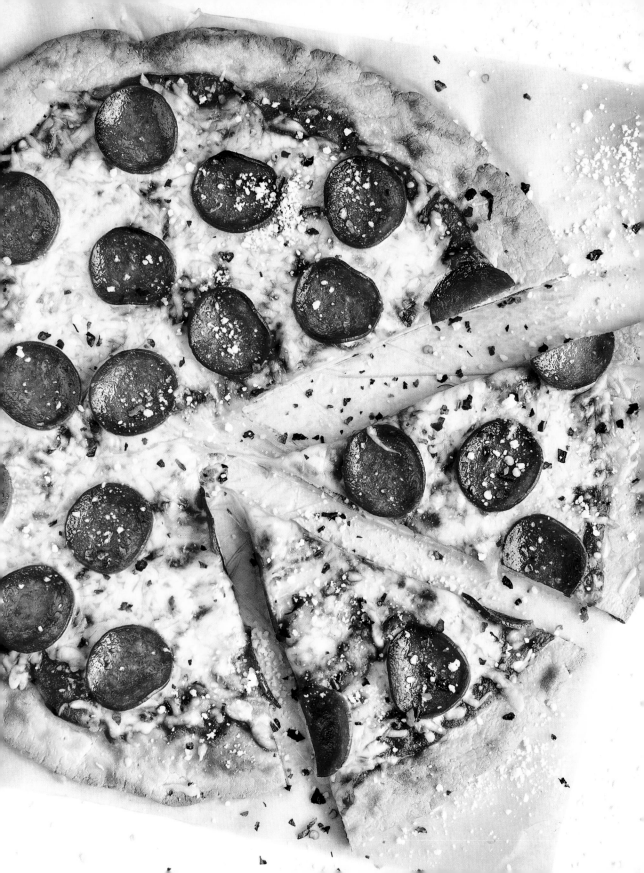

FATHEAD PIZZA CRUST

If there is one keto recipe that surprises people the most, fathead pizza crust is it. I make this pizza crust almost every week so I can just add toppings and whip up a quick pizza dinner. My kids gobble it up eagerly, and my (not all keto!) friends and family can never tell this crust is keto-friendly—it's a true replacement for the real thing.

1 recipe Fathead Dough
  (page 17)

MAKES 8 SERVINGS

SERVING SIZE
1 slice, or ⅛ of entire crust

PER SERVING
ALMOND FLOUR VERSION
144 calories
12 g fat
3 g total carbs
2 g net carbs
8 g protein

COCONUT FLOUR VERSION
117 calories
8 g fat
4 g total carbs
2 g net carbs
7 g protein

1. Preheat the oven to 400°F. If using a pizza stone, preheat it inside the oven at the same time.

2. Make the dough through Step 2 of the instructions on pages 17 to 19.

3. Place the dough between two greased pieces of parchment paper and roll out to a ⅛- to ⅓-inch thickness, depending on your preference.

4. Lift the bottom piece of parchment paper. Use a toothpick or fork to poke lots of holes throughout the crust to prevent bubbling.

5. Slide the parchment paper with the crust onto a pizza pan or pizza stone.

6. Bake for 6 minutes. Poke more holes in any places where you see bubbles forming and rotate the pizza stone or pan. Bake for 3 to 8 more minutes, depending on thickness, until golden brown.

TIPS & VARIATIONS • To make pizza, add sauce and desired toppings to the prebaked crust and return to the oven for about 10 minutes, until the cheese melts and toppings cook to your desired liking. For the crispiest crust, bake directly on the rack, or place on the pizza stone without parchment paper.

• You can adjust the texture by changing the thickness. A thicker crust will be softer and chewier; a thinner crust will be crispier.

• Get a pizza stone if you can! It significantly improves the texture.

• For more Italian flavor, add ½ teaspoon garlic powder and ½ tablespoon Italian seasoning to the dough.

ONE-PAN MEALS

15-MINUTE EGG ROLL IN A BOWL

Stir-fry was one of the first meals I learned to cook on my own. When I moved out of my parents' house, dinner on most nights was a mishmash of ingredients out of a wok. These days I'm much more intentional about the flavors that go into my stir-fry, but it's still one of my favorite low carb meals. This one is super simple and takes just 15 minutes to prepare!

1. In a large sauté pan, heat the avocado oil over medium-high heat. Add the garlic and ginger and sauté about 1 minute, until fragrant.

2. Add the ground beef, season with sea salt and black pepper, and cook until browned, 7 to 10 minutes.

3. Reduce the heat to medium. Add the coleslaw mix and coconut aminos and stir to coat. Cover and cook for about 5 minutes, or until the cabbage is tender.

4. Remove from heat. Stir in the sesame oil and green onions.

TIPS & VARIATIONS • This recipe uses shredded coleslaw mix for convenience. If you prefer, you can shred about ½ head of cabbage yourself instead.

• Toasted sesame oil has a low smoke point, so don't add it until after removing the pan from the heat.

• If you like a bit of heat, try adding some red pepper flakes.

1 *tablespoon* avocado oil

4 *cloves* garlic, minced

3 *tablespoons* minced or grated fresh ginger, or ¾ teaspoon ground ginger

1 *pound* ground beef

1 *teaspoon* sea salt

¼ *teaspoon* black pepper (or more if you want it spicy)

6 *cups (~1 pound)* shredded coleslaw mix

¼ *cup* coconut aminos

2 *teaspoons* toasted sesame oil

¼ *cup (0.9 ounce)* thinly sliced green onions

MAKES 6 SERVINGS

SERVING SIZE
1 cup (~5.5 ounces)

PER SERVING
231 calories
15 g fat
8 g total carbs
4 g net carbs
15 g protein

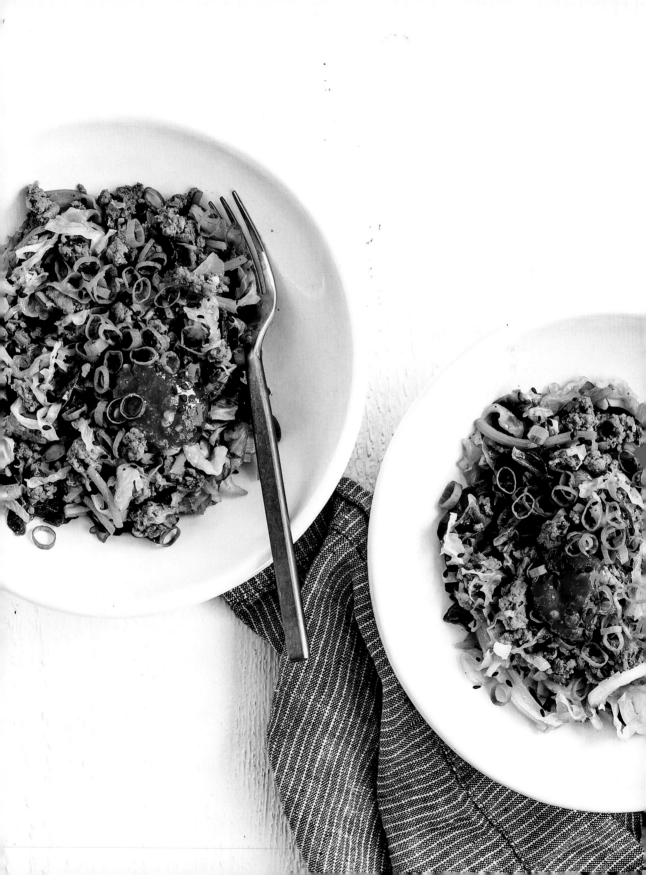

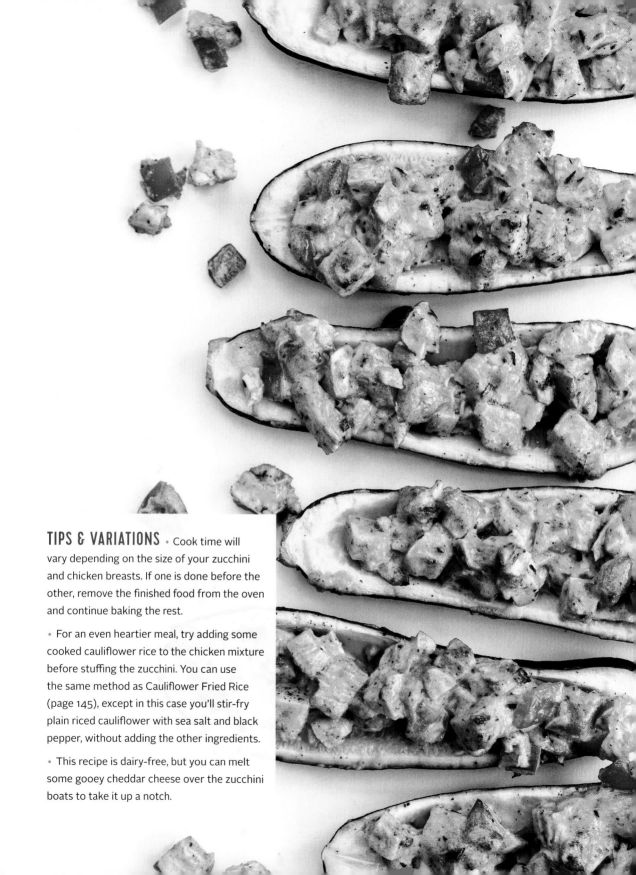

TIPS & VARIATIONS • Cook time will vary depending on the size of your zucchini and chicken breasts. If one is done before the other, remove the finished food from the oven and continue baking the rest.

• For an even heartier meal, try adding some cooked cauliflower rice to the chicken mixture before stuffing the zucchini. You can use the same method as Cauliflower Fried Rice (page 145), except in this case you'll stir-fry plain riced cauliflower with sea salt and black pepper, without adding the other ingredients.

• This recipe is dairy-free, but you can melt some gooey cheddar cheese over the zucchini boats to take it up a notch.

CAJUN CHICKEN ZUCCHINI BOATS

I've never been to Louisiana, but I do love Cajun spices! This recipe incorporates all the best things about Cajun chicken, stuffed into zucchini to up your veggie intake and make a complete meal. It's light on carbs and calories yet brimming with flavor.

1. Preheat the oven to 450°F. Line a 20 × 14-inch sheet pan or two 14 × 10-inch sheet pans with parchment paper.

2. Halve the zucchini lengthwise. Use a spoon to scoop out a well in each zucchini half. (Save the leftover flesh for another use.)

3. Place the zucchini, cut side up, on one side of the large sheet pan. Place the bell pepper in the middle of the pan. Place the chicken on the other side, so that the chicken breasts are not touching each other or the veggies. (If using two pans, place the zucchini on one, the chicken and bell peppers on the other.)

4. Drizzle the zucchini and peppers with some avocado oil, then brush both sides of the chicken with oil. Season the zucchini, peppers, and chicken with the sea salt and black pepper.

5. Transfer the pan(s) to the oven and bake for 15 to 20 minutes, until the chicken is cooked through and the peppers and zucchini are soft. Leave the oven on. Set the sheet pan(s) aside until the chicken is cool enough to handle.

6. Meanwhile, in a large bowl, whisk together the mayonnaise, thyme, smoked paprika, garlic powder, oregano, and cayenne pepper (start with ¼ teaspoon cayenne and adjust to taste).

7. When cool enough to handle, cut the cooked chicken into bite-size pieces. Add the chicken and bell peppers to the bowl with the mayonnaise mixture, and stir to coat.

8. Pat the zucchini dry with paper towels. Stuff the chicken mixture into the zucchini boats. Return to the oven for 5 to 10 minutes, until hot.

4 *medium* zucchini (6 ounces each)

1 *large (7-ounce)* bell pepper, coarsely chopped

1 *pound* boneless, skinless chicken breast

⅓ *cup* avocado oil

1 *teaspoon* sea salt

½ *teaspoon* black pepper

1 *cup* 2-Minute Avocado Oil Mayonnaise (page 235)

2 *teaspoons* fresh thyme, finely chopped

1 *teaspoon* smoked paprika

½ *teaspoon* garlic powder

½ *teaspoon* dried oregano

½ *teaspoon* cayenne pepper, or to taste

MAKES 8 SERVINGS

SERVING SIZE

1 stuffed zucchini boat (4 ounces)

PER SERVING

373 calories
32 g fat
4 g total carbs
3 g net carbs
14 g protein

ONE-PAN MEALS

TUSCAN GARLIC CHICKEN CASSEROLE

Casseroles are classic American fare, but they were foreign to me growing up in a Russian household. That was all the more reason to fall in love with them as an adult! Casseroles offer so many conveniences for busy families: They are easy to prepare in advance, freeze beautifully, and eliminate the need for a side dish. This one transforms juicy, Tuscan garlic chicken into the ultimate comfort food.

1. Preheat the oven to 400°F.

2. In a large saucepan, heat the butter over medium heat. Add the garlic and sauté for about 1 minute, until fragrant.

3. Add the cream, chicken broth, and Italian seasoning. Bring to a simmer, then simmer gently for about 10 minutes, or until thick enough to coat the back of a spoon.

4. Meanwhile, in a large bowl, stir together the shredded chicken, spinach, and sun-dried tomatoes.

5. When the sauce has thickened a bit in the saucepan, reduce the heat to low and don't let it simmer or boil. Whisk in the grated Parmesan gradually, ⅓ cup at a time, until smooth. Season with sea salt and black pepper, to taste.

6. Stir the sauce into the bowl with the chicken and spinach.

7. Transfer the casserole mixture to a glass or ceramic 8-inch square baking dish. Sprinkle with mozzarella.

8. Bake for 10 to 20 minutes, until the casserole is hot and the cheese starts to brown.

TIPS & VARIATIONS • If you don't have sun-dried tomatoes or want to reduce carbs, try roasted or sautéed red peppers instead.

• For a pop of color, garnish with spinach or fresh parsley.

• This is a great make-ahead meal. You can assemble it and refrigerate or freeze, then bake right before serving.

1 *tablespoon* butter

6 *cloves* garlic, minced

1 *cup* heavy cream

¼ *cup* chicken broth

1 *tablespoon* Italian seasoning

1 *pound (~3 cups)* shredded chicken (rotisserie, or cooked from 1⅓ pounds raw)

1 *(12-ounce) bag* frozen spinach, thawed, drained, and squeezed dry

½ *cup* chopped sun-dried tomatoes

⅔ *cup (2.7 ounces)* grated Parmesan cheese

½ *teaspoon* sea salt, or to taste

¼ *teaspoon* black pepper, or to taste

1 *cup (4 ounces)* shredded mozzarella cheese

MAKES 6 SERVINGS

SERVING SIZE
1 cup (~6 ounces)

PER SERVING
430 calories
29 g fat
11 g total carbs
8 g net carbs
32 g protein

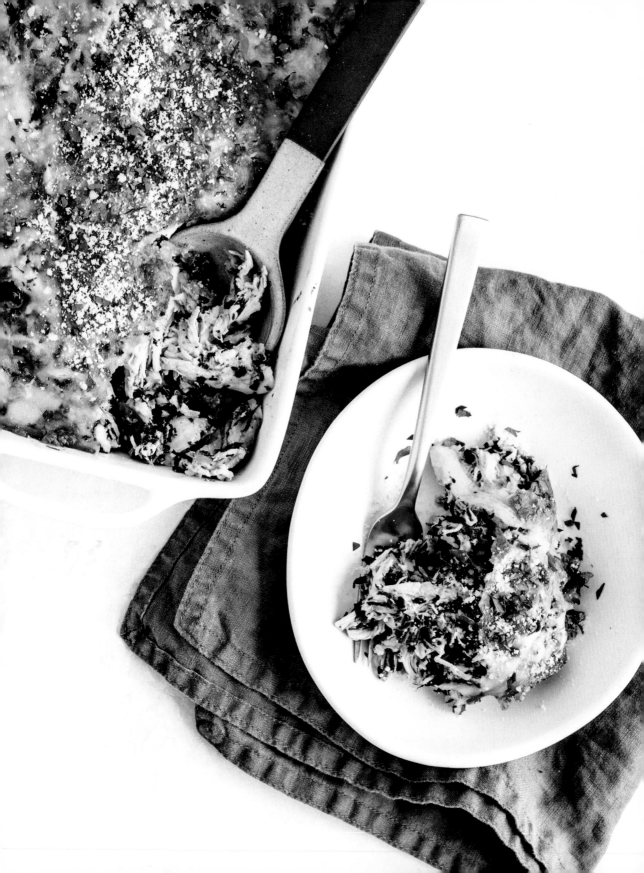

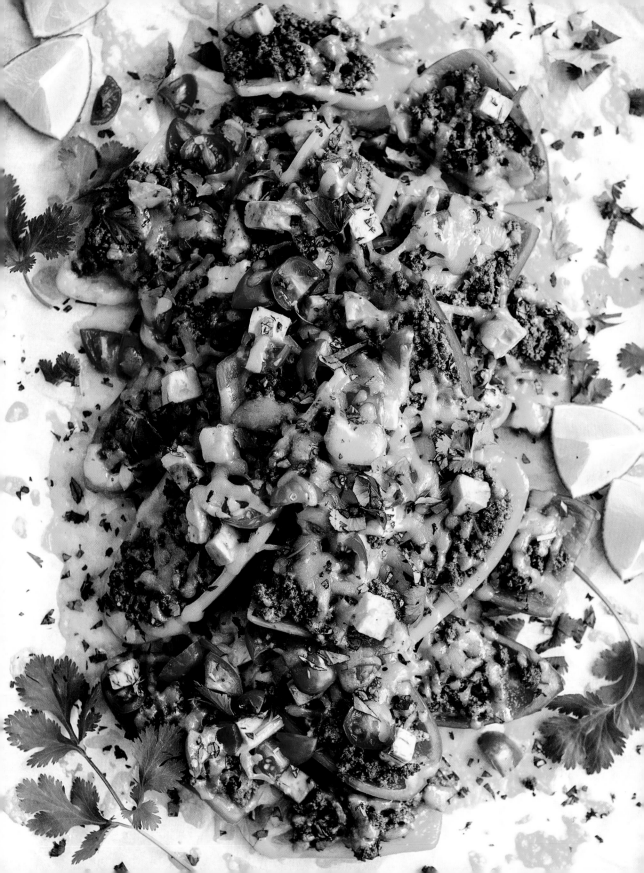

MINI BELL PEPPER NACHOS

Dinner on the table in about 20 minutes—what could be better? This dish offers everything you love about nachos but replaces the carb-filled chips with nutritious, naturally sweet bell peppers. You can serve these as an appetizer, but they are also filling enough for a meal.

1. Preheat the oven to 450°F. Line a 20 × 14-inch sheet pan or two 14 × 10-inch sheet pans with foil or parchment paper.

2. In a sauté pan, heat the oil over medium-high heat. Add the ground beef and stir-fry for 7 to 10 minutes, breaking apart with a spatula, until browned.

3. Add the taco seasoning and ½ cup water. Stir-fry for a couple more minutes, until most of the water is absorbed or evaporated.

4. Arrange the peppers in a single layer on the pan(s), cut side up. Fill with the taco meat. Top with the tomatoes and avocado, then the cheddar.

5. Place the peppers in the oven for 5 to 8 minutes, until the cheese melts. Sprinkle with cilantro to serve.

1 tablespoon avocado oil

1 pound ground beef

2 tablespoons Taco Seasoning (page 239)

1 pound (about 20) mini bell peppers, halved lengthwise and seeds removed

¾ cup (5 ounces) finely diced tomatoes

1 medium (6-ounce) avocado, finely diced

2 cups (8 ounces) shredded cheddar cheese

2 tablespoons chopped fresh cilantro

MAKES 8 SERVINGS

SERVING SIZE
5 stuffed mini pepper halves (~3.5 ounces)

PER SERVING
374 calories
27 g fat
6 g total carbs
4 g net carbs
24 g protein

TIPS & VARIATIONS · Mini bell peppers are available at most grocery stores. However, if you can't find them, you can slice large bell peppers into wide boats for a similar effect.

· Traditional nacho toppings like onions, sour cream, a squeeze of lime, or hot sauce make great additions. Avoid higher-carb ingredients such as beans and corn.

· This recipe also works well with shredded beef, chicken, or even pork instead of ground beef.

ONE-PAN MEALS

SPAGHETTI SQUASH BOLOGNESE

Spaghetti was one of the hardest things for me to give up when I went keto—so I didn't! You can easily make your favorite pasta dishes keto-friendly by using spaghetti squash or zucchini noodles in place of carb-heavy pasta. This meal is super simple to make and you'll feel like you're eating your favorite pasta dish!

1. Preheat the oven to 425°F. Line a baking sheet with foil and grease lightly.

2. **Make the spaghetti squash:** Use a sharp chef's knife to slice the spaghetti squash in half. To make it easier, use the knife to score where you'll be cutting first, then slice. Cut crosswise for longer noodles or lengthwise for shorter ones. Scoop out the seeds. Drizzle the insides of the spaghetti squash halves with the avocado oil. Season with sea salt.

3. Place the spaghetti squash halves cut side down on the lined baking sheet. Roast for 25 to 35 minutes, until the skin pierces easily with a knife. The knife should be able to go in pretty deep with just very slight resistance.

4. **Meanwhile, make the Bolognese sauce:** In a sauté pan, heat the oil over medium-high heat. Add the garlic and sauté for about 1 minute, until fragrant. Add the ground beef, season with sea salt and black pepper, and cook for 7 to 10 minutes, breaking apart with a spatula, until browned. Add the marinara sauce, bring to a simmer, and simmer for 10 minutes.

5. When the squash is done, remove from the oven and let the squash rest on the pan for 10 minutes. Then use a fork to release the strands.

6. Add the squash strands to the pan with the meat sauce and toss to coat. Adjust sea salt and black pepper to taste if needed.

7. To serve, divide among 6 plates. Sprinkle each serving with 2 tablespoons Parmesan, if using, and 1 teaspoon parsley.

SPAGHETTI SQUASH

- 1 large (3-pound) spaghetti squash
- 1 tablespoon avocado oil
- ½ teaspoon sea salt

BOLOGNESE SAUCE

- 1 tablespoon avocado oil
- 4 cloves garlic, minced
- 1 pound ground beef
- 1 teaspoon sea salt, plus more to taste
- ¼ teaspoon black pepper, plus more to taste
- 1½ cups marinara sauce, no sugar added

SERVING

- ¾ cup (3 ounces) grated Parmesan cheese (omit for dairy-free)
- 2 tablespoons chopped fresh parsley

MAKES 6 SERVINGS

SERVING SIZE
1 cup

PER SERVING
430 calories
28 g fat
17 g total carbs
14 g net carbs
28 g protein

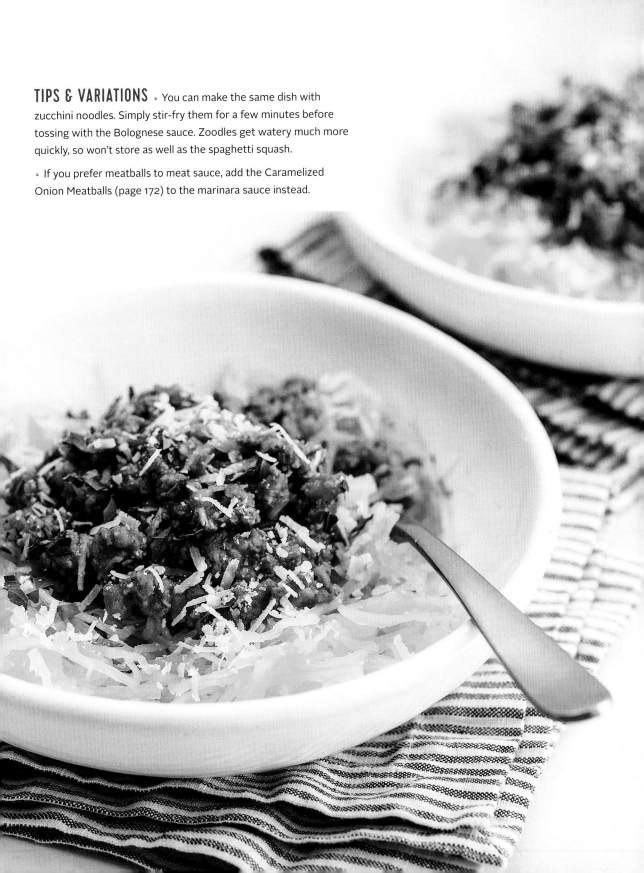

TIPS & VARIATIONS • You can make the same dish with zucchini noodles. Simply stir-fry them for a few minutes before tossing with the Bolognese sauce. Zoodles get watery much more quickly, so won't store as well as the spaghetti squash.

• If you prefer meatballs to meat sauce, add the Caramelized Onion Meatballs (page 172) to the marinara sauce instead.

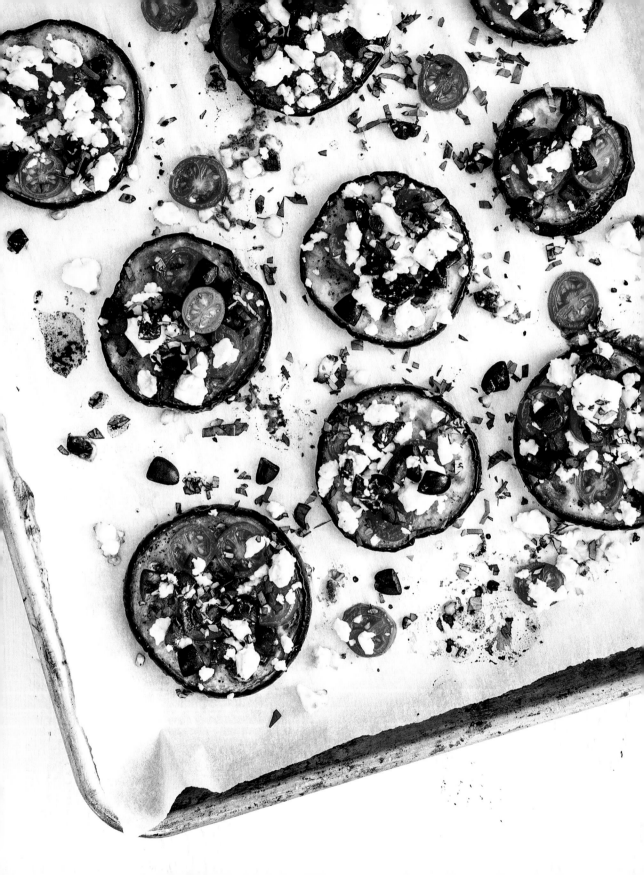

MEDITERRANEAN EGGPLANT PIZZAS

Eggplant pizzas are simply pizzas made with eggplant rounds instead of the crust. You can certainly make them with traditional marinara and pepperoni, but this recipe has a Mediterranean flair instead. It's chock-full of Greek flavors and happens to be vegetarian, too!

2 medium (1-pound) eggplant, cut crosswise into slices ½ inch thick

¼ cup olive oil

2 teaspoons sea salt

½ teaspoon black pepper

½ cup Basic Greek Vinaigrette (page 251)

2 cups (10.6 ounces) grape tomatoes, sliced into circles

½ cup (2.5 ounces) Kalamata olives, pitted and thinly sliced

1⅓ cup (7 ounces) crumbled feta cheese (omit for dairy-free)

¼ cup fresh basil, cut into ribbons

1. Preheat the oven to 400°F. Line an extra-large baking sheet, at least 20 × 14 inches in size (or two 10 × 14-inch pans) with parchment paper.

2. Place the eggplant slices in a single layer on the lined baking sheet(s) and brush both sides with the oil. Season both sides with sea salt and black pepper.

3. Bake for 25 to 30 minutes, until the eggplant is soft and golden.

4. Spread about 1 teaspoon Greek salad dressing on each eggplant slice. Top each eggplant piece with 2 to 4 tomato slices and 2 or 3 olive slices. Sprinkle each with ½ tablespoon crumbled feta.

5. Return to the oven and bake for 5 to 10 minutes, until the tomatoes are soft. Sprinkle with fresh basil before serving.

MAKES 6 SERVINGS

SERVING SIZE

4 mini pizzas in varying sizes (8 ounces)

PER SERVING

341 calories

29 g fat

12 g total carbs

6 g net carbs

6 g protein

TIPS & VARIATIONS • You can easily substitute marinara sauce or pesto for the Greek salad dressing in this recipe.

• To meal prep this recipe, you can roast the eggplant rounds and chop the toppings ahead of time. Simply assemble and finish baking the day of.

ONE-PAN MEALS

CHICKEN-BROCCOLI ALFREDO CASSEROLE

When I used to eat real pasta, fettuccine Alfredo was my number one choice. You can totally use the sauce from this recipe over zoodles or spaghetti squash as a side dish, but this time I used it for a whole meal. This casserole is the ultimate keto comfort food. No noodles needed!

1. Preheat the oven to 400°F. Line a 20 × 14-inch baking sheet or two 14 × 10-inch pans, with foil or parchment paper.

2. **Prepare the chicken and broccoli:** Place the chicken breasts on one side of the pan, 1 inch apart, and broccoli and bell peppers on the other. Drizzle all over with melted butter, including both sides of the chicken. Season with sea salt and black pepper.

3. Roast the chicken, broccoli, and peppers for 20 to 25 minutes, until the chicken is cooked through and the broccoli is tender.

4. **Meanwhile, make the Alfredo sauce:** In a large sauté pan, melt the butter over medium heat. Add the garlic and sauté for about 1 minute, until fragrant.

5. Add the cream. Bring to a gentle simmer, then continue to simmer for 5 to 7 minutes, until the sauce begins to thicken and the volume is reduced by about one-third.

6. Reduce heat to low. Gradually whisk in the Parmesan and keep whisking over low heat, until smooth. Stir in sea salt and black pepper to taste, if needed. Cover to keep warm and set aside.

7. When the chicken and broccoli are done, remove the pan from the oven but leave it on. Let the chicken cool slightly.

8. Chop the chicken. In a large bowl, toss it with the broccoli, peppers, and Alfredo sauce.

9. Transfer the mixture to a 9 × 13-inch glass baking dish. Sprinkle the mozzarella evenly on top. Bake for about 10 minutes, or until the cheese on top is melted and browned.

CHICKEN AND BROCCOLI

- 1½ *pounds* boneless, skinless chicken breasts
- 1½ *pounds (~12 cups)* broccoli florets
- 1 *large (7-ounce)* bell pepper, cut into 2-inch pieces
- 4 *tablespoons (½ stick)* butter, melted
- 1 *teaspoon* sea salt
- ¼ *teaspoon* black pepper

ALFREDO SAUCE

- 1 *tablespoon* butter
- 6 *cloves* garlic, minced
- 1½ *cups* heavy cream
- ½ *cup (2 ounces)* grated Parmesan cheese

  Sea salt and black pepper

ASSEMBLY

- 2 *cups (8 ounces)* shredded mozzarella cheese

MAKES 8 SERVINGS

SERVING SIZE
1 cup (~7 ounces)

PER SERVING
467 calories
33 g fat
9 g total carbs
7 g net carbs
31 g protein

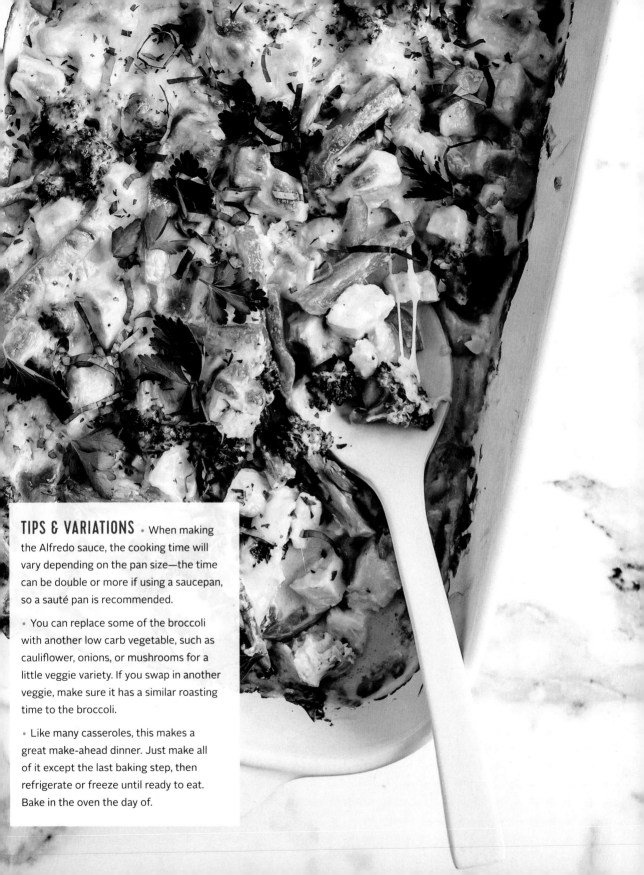

TIPS & VARIATIONS • When making the Alfredo sauce, the cooking time will vary depending on the pan size—the time can be double or more if using a saucepan, so a sauté pan is recommended.

• You can replace some of the broccoli with another low carb vegetable, such as cauliflower, onions, or mushrooms for a little veggie variety. If you swap in another veggie, make sure it has a similar roasting time to the broccoli.

• Like many casseroles, this makes a great make-ahead dinner. Just make all of it except the last baking step, then refrigerate or freeze until ready to eat. Bake in the oven the day of.

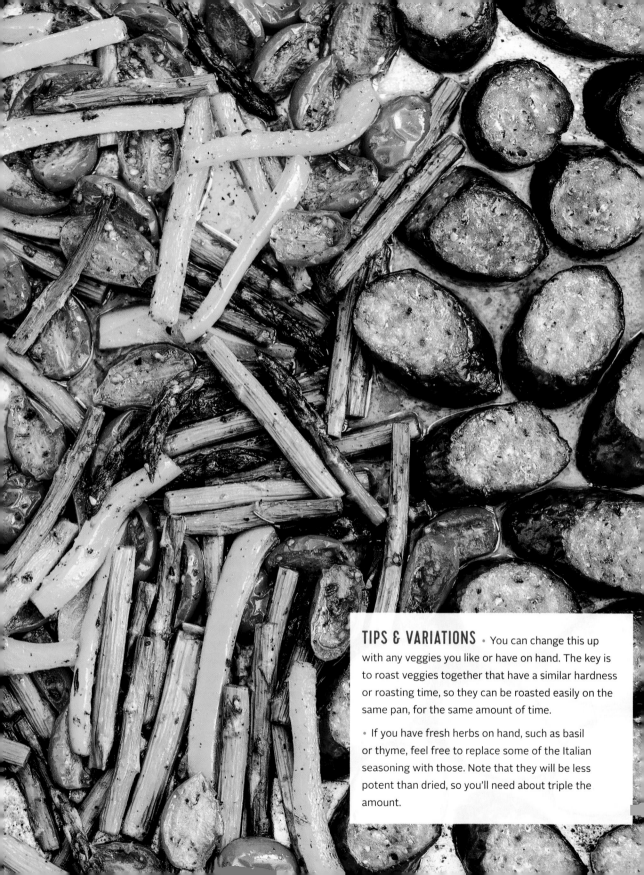

TIPS & VARIATIONS • You can change this up with any veggies you like or have on hand. The key is to roast veggies together that have a similar hardness or roasting time, so they can be roasted easily on the same pan, for the same amount of time.

• If you have fresh herbs on hand, such as basil or thyme, feel free to replace some of the Italian seasoning with those. Note that they will be less potent than dried, so you'll need about triple the amount.

KIELBASA VEGGIE SHEET PAN DINNER

If "quick and easy" is your jam (like it is mine!), you *need* to add sheet pan dinners to your repertoire. Cooking meat and veggies side by side on a single pan means less time, less stress, and less cleanup. And kielbasa provides a nice variation over the usual chicken and beef protein options.

1. Preheat the oven to 400°F. Line a 20 × 14-inch baking sheet or two 14 × 10-inch pans with foil and grease well.

2. Arrange the kielbasa in a single layer on the baking sheet. Roast for 12 to 15 minutes, until it starts to brown on the bottom.

3. Meanwhile, in a large bowl, toss together the veggies.

4. In a small bowl, whisk together the oil, sea salt, Italian seasoning, paprika, garlic powder, and black pepper. Pour over the veggies and toss to coat.

5. When the kielbasa is done, remove the pan from the oven but leave it on. Flip the kielbasa pieces over and move them to one side of the pan, leaving space for the veggies.

6. Arrange the veggies in a single layer on the other side of the extra-large pan, or on the second pan if using two pans. Roast for 18 to 20 minutes, until the veggies are tender and the kielbasa is further browned.

1½ pounds kielbasa, cut on the diagonal into ½-inch-thick slices (~6½ cups)

1 pound asparagus, trimmed, cut into 2-inch pieces (~3 cups)

1½ cups (8 ounces) grape tomatoes, halved

1 large orange bell pepper, cut into 2-inch pieces (~1½ cups)

3 tablespoons olive oil

1 teaspoon sea salt

1 teaspoon Italian seasoning

1 teaspoon paprika

½ teaspoon garlic powder

¼ teaspoon black pepper

MAKES 8 CUPS (4 SERVINGS)

SERVING SIZE
2 cups (~8.8 ounces)

PER SERVING
686 calories
59 g fat
10 g total carbs
7 g net carbs
26 g protein

ONE-PAN MEALS

PAN-FRIED BAJA FISH TACOS

There's a reason Minnesota is called the land of 10,000 lakes—it's where Minnesotans spend their summers! And we have some great fish taco joints at the lake, but I stick to my keto lifestyle and skip the tortillas. I've mastered the perfect keto-friendly tortilla so I can make my own fish tacos at home. These tacos taste just like the real thing and conjure up memories of summers at the lake.

1. **Marinate the fish:** In a medium bowl, whisk together the oil, lime juice, and taco seasoning. Add the cod pieces and mix with your hands, coating well. Cover and refrigerate for 15 minutes.

2. **Make the taco sauce:** In a small bowl, whisk together the mayonnaise, lime juice, and taco seasoning until smooth.

3. **Prepare the tacos:** When the fish is done marinating, in a large skillet, heat the oil over medium-high heat. Shake any excess marinade from the fish pieces and add to the pan in a single layer. Cook for 2 to 3 minutes, until browned on the bottom. Flip and cook the other side, until opaque and browned.

4. Warm the prepared fathead tortillas in the oven or microwave, to make them pliable. Cover to keep warm as you assemble the tacos one at a time (they must stay warm to be flexible).

5. To assemble the fish tacos, place 2 ounces (⅛ of the total amount) of the fish inside a fathead tortilla. Add the tomatoes, avocado, red cabbage, and cilantro. Drizzle with the taco sauce.

MARINATED FISH

- ¼ cup olive oil
- 2 tablespoons lime juice
- ¾ teaspoon Taco Seasoning (page 239)
- 1 pound cod, cut into 1½-inch pieces

TACO SAUCE

- ⅓ cup 2-Minute Avocado Oil Mayonnaise (page 235)
- 1 tablespoon lime juice
- ¾ teaspoon Taco Seasoning (page 239)

TACOS

- 1 tablespoon olive oil
- 8 (6-inch) Pliable Fathead Tortillas (page 201)
- 1 cup (8 ounces) diced tomatoes
- 1 medium (6-ounce) avocado, diced
- 1 cup (3.5 ounces) shredded red cabbage
- ½ cup chopped fresh cilantro

MAKES 4 SERVINGS

SERVING SIZE
2 fish tacos (~14.5 ounces)

PER SERVING
ALMOND FLOUR VERSION
603 calories
50 g fat
10 g total carbs
5 g net carbs
29 g protein

COCONUT FLOUR VERSION
575 calories
46 g fat
11 g total carbs
6 g net carbs
28 g protein

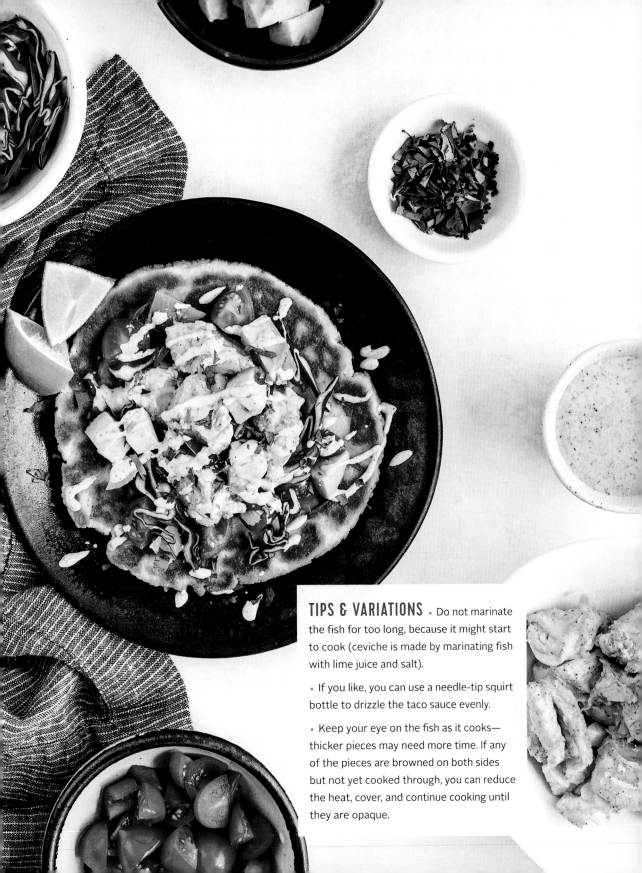

TIPS & VARIATIONS • Do not marinate the fish for too long, because it might start to cook (ceviche is made by marinating fish with lime juice and salt).

• If you like, you can use a needle-tip squirt bottle to drizzle the taco sauce evenly.

• Keep your eye on the fish as it cooks—thicker pieces may need more time. If any of the pieces are browned on both sides but not yet cooked through, you can reduce the heat, cover, and continue cooking until they are opaque.

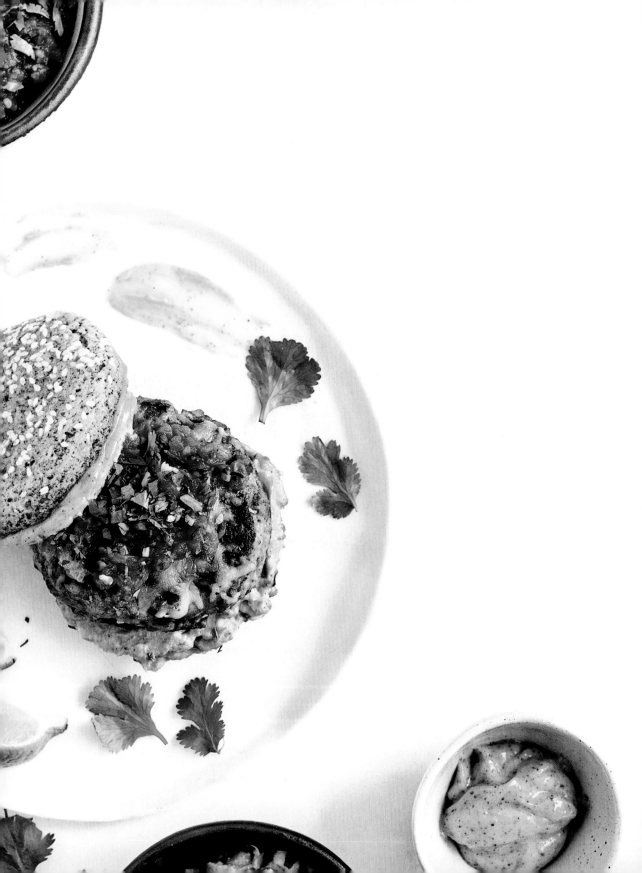

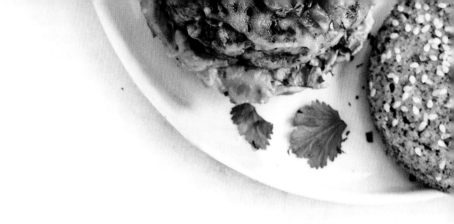

MEAT & FISH ENTRÉES

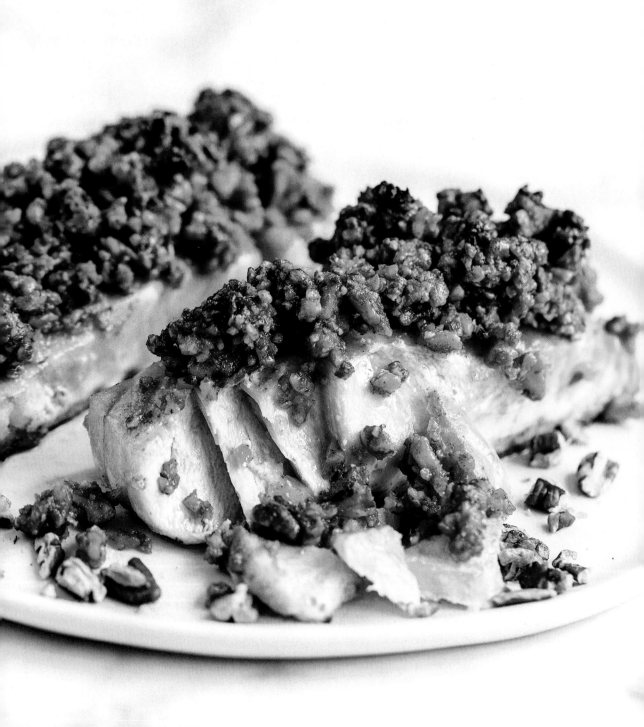

MAPLE PECAN-CRUSTED SALMON

Salmon contains plenty of healthy omega-3 fats, making it an excellent protein choice for the keto lifestyle. It's a flavorful fish on its own but pairs particularly well with sweet flavors, like maple or honey. Keto guidelines don't permit these sugar-y sweeteners, but we can create our own keto-friendly marinade glaze with maple extract, butter, and a natural sugar-free sweetener. The pecan crust on this fish is sweet, smoky, and rich, all at the same time.

1. Preheat the oven to 400°F. Line a large baking sheet with foil.

2. Arrange the salmon fillets on the lined baking sheet.

3. In a medium bowl, make the maple glaze. Whisk together the melted butter, powdered erythritol, maple extract, smoked paprika, sea salt, and cayenne pepper.

4. Brush both sides of the salmon with the maple glaze, using about half of it. Set the remaining glaze aside.

5. Pulse the pecans in a food processor until finely chopped. Don't overmix or it will turn into pecan flour. (Alternatively, chop with a knife.) Add the chopped pecans to the remaining glaze and stir together to coat.

6. Spoon the pecan mixture evenly over the salmon fillets, pressing on the top with your hands.

7. Bake for 9 to 12 minutes, until the fish flakes easily with a fork.

4 *salmon* fillets (4 ounces each)

4 *tablespoons (½ stick)* butter, melted

2 *tablespoons* powdered erythritol

½ *teaspoon* real maple extract

½ *teaspoon* smoked paprika

½ *teaspoon* sea salt

¼ *teaspoon* cayenne pepper, or less if you prefer a milder marinade

¾ *cup* pecans

MAKES 4 SERVINGS

SERVING SIZE

1 salmon fillet (4 ounces) with nut topping

PER SERVING

392 calories
32 g fat
7 g total carbs
1 g net carbs
24 g protein

TIPS & VARIATIONS • If you don't have pecans, other types of nuts, such as walnuts or almonds, will also work.

• This recipe makes a lightly sweet topping. If you like it very sweet, you can double the sweetener. Conversely, if you prefer not to use a sweetener, you can omit it.

WHITE WINE SEARED CHICKEN BREASTS

Not all recipes have to be adapted to be keto—many dishes fit into the lifestyle naturally. This white wine seared chicken breast is a great example. You can make it using simple ingredients found at any grocery store. With its quick prep time and fancy feel, it happens to be versatile for many occasions—for date night or for company!

1. Season the chicken on both sides with sea salt and black pepper.

2. In a large skillet or sauté pan, melt 1 tablespoon of the butter over medium-high heat. Add the chicken and sauté for 5 to 8 minutes per side, until cooked through and browned.

3. Remove the chicken from the pan and cover with foil.

4. Add another 1 tablespoon butter to the pan. Add the garlic and shallot, and sauté for about 1 minute, until fragrant.

5. Add the wine and broth to the pan and use a wooden spoon to scrape any browned bits from the bottom. Bring to a gentle boil, then lower the heat and simmer for about 7 to 8 minutes, until the liquid volume is reduced by half.

6. Reduce the heat to low. Stir in the remaining 2 tablespoons butter, parsley, and thyme, just until the butter melts.

7. Serve the sauce over the chicken.

TIPS & VARIATIONS • Do not move the chicken around in the pan. Let it cook without moving to get nice and brown.

• Be careful not to burn the butter when sautéing the chicken. If you find that the butter is burning easily, you can also swap in avocado oil.

• For best results, make sure the broth and wine mixture reduces and thickens before adding the final 2 pats of butter. If you add the butter early by mistake, simmer gently to thicken it more.

• For a richer pan sauce that's also nutrient-packed, replace regular chicken broth with chicken bone broth.

4 *medium* boneless, skinless chicken breasts (8 ounces each)

1 *teaspoon* sea salt

¼ *teaspoon* black pepper

4 *tablespoons* (½ *stick*) butter, cut into 1-tablespoon pats

2 *cloves* garlic, minced

1 *medium (2.5-ounce)* shallot, finely chopped

½ *cup* white cooking wine

½ *cup* chicken broth

½ *tablespoon* chopped fresh parsley

½ *tablespoon* fresh thyme, chopped

MAKES 4 SERVINGS

SERVING SIZE
1 chicken breast (8 ounces) with 2 to 3 tablespoons sauce (depending on how much you reduce it)

PER SERVING
288 calories
14 g fat
2 g total carbs
2 g net carbs
29 g protein

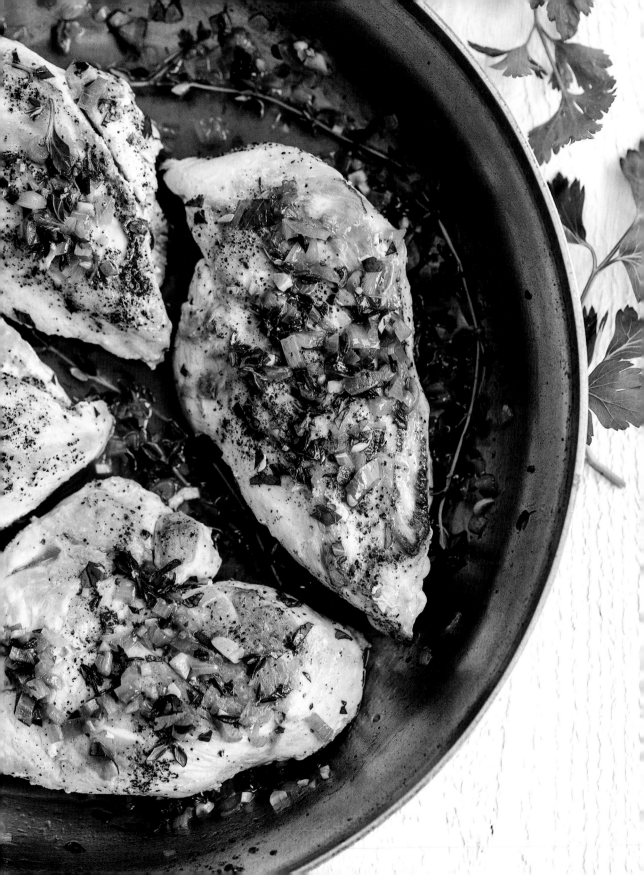

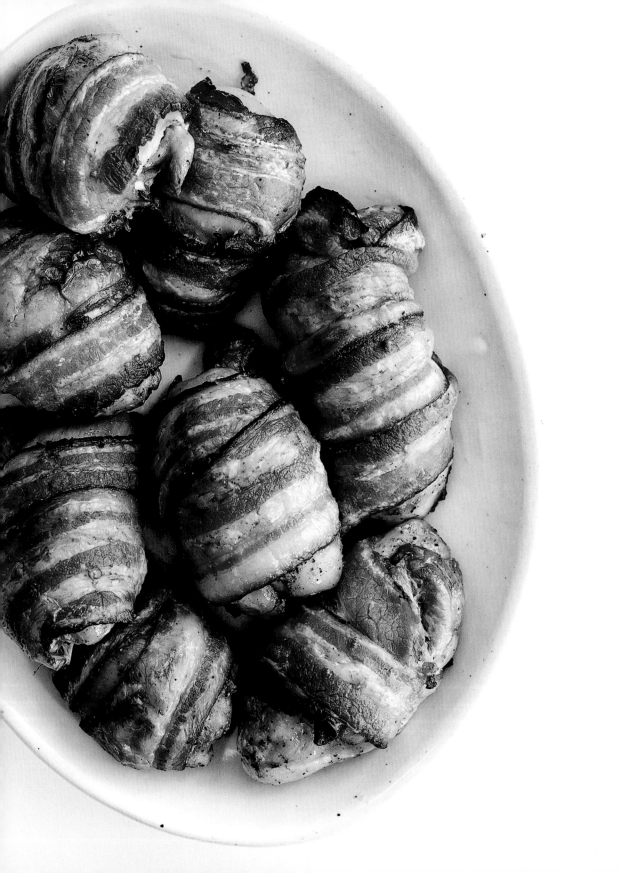

BACON-WRAPPED CHICKEN THIGHS

I *love* chicken. It is definitely my protein of choice, and clearly many of my readers agree—the chicken recipes on Wholesome Yum are very popular! But on a keto diet, it can be hard to get a good fat/protein ratio with only lean chicken breasts. I still find ways to enjoy them (and this book is filled with them!), but chicken thighs are a great higher-fat alternative. And wrapping them in smoky bacon? Perfection.

8 *medium* boneless, skinless chicken thighs (~2.5 ounces each)

¼ *cup* avocado oil

½ *teaspoon* paprika

1 *teaspoon* sea salt

¼ *teaspoon* black pepper

8 *slices* bacon

MAKES 4 SERVINGS

SERVING SIZE
2 wrapped chicken thighs (~6 ounces)

PER SERVING
606 calories
52 g fat
0 g total carbs
0 g net carbs
30 g protein

1. Preheat the oven to 450°F. Line a sheet pan with foil.

2. Place the chicken thighs in a single layer on the baking sheet so that they don't touch each other.

3. Brush the chicken on both sides with the oil. Season with paprika, sea salt, and black pepper.

4. Wrap each chicken thigh tightly in a slice of bacon, tucking the end underneath to secure it. Place seam side down on the baking sheet.

5. Roast for 18 to 22 minutes, until the chicken is almost or just barely cooked through. Remove from the oven and drain any liquid from the pan.

6. Move the oven rack to the top. Switch the oven to broil and place the chicken under the broiler for 2 to 3 minutes, until the bacon is crispy.

TIPS & VARIATIONS • For even crispier bacon, roast the chicken thighs on a wire rack set over a sheet pan. This provides more air circulation, and some of the bacon fat drips down, allowing the bacon to crisp up. While we need plenty of fat on a keto diet, losing a little bit of it to make crispier bacon is well worth it!

• Feel free to add any other herbs and spices you like. A teaspoon of Italian seasoning on the chicken works well, as does a sprinkle of grated Parmesan cheese over the bacon.

MEAT & FISH ENTRÉES

SLOW COOKER CREAMY SALSA CHICKEN

We all have days when we don't have time to make dinner. If you know that in advance, throwing something into the slow cooker in the morning is a great option. This easy salsa chicken needs just four ingredients and about 5 minutes of prep time. It doesn't get any easier than that!

4 *boneless,* skinless chicken breasts (6 ounces each)

1 *cup* Pantry Staple Salsa (page 240)

3 *ounces (6 tablespoons)* cream cheese

1 *cup (4 ounces)* shredded pepper jack cheese

MAKES 4 SERVINGS

1. Place the chicken breasts in a slow cooker and pour the salsa over them. Cook on low for 6 to 8 hours or on high for 3 to 4 hours, until the chicken is cooked through and tender.

2. Close to serving time, heat the cream cheese in the microwave for about 30 seconds, or let it sit at room temperature to soften.

3. Remove the chicken from the slow cooker and set aside, scraping any excess salsa to leave it in the slow cooker. Whisk the cream cheese in the slow cooker until the sauce is smooth.

4. Return the chicken to the slow cooker and sprinkle the pepper jack over it. Cover and keep the heat on for 10 to 15 minutes, until the cheese melts.

5. Spoon the creamy salsa mixture over the chicken to serve.

SERVING SIZE

1 chicken breast (~6 ounces) with 2 ounces sauce

PER SERVING

350 calories
18 g fat
5 g total carbs
5 g net carbs
36 g protein

TIPS & VARIATIONS • If you prefer less spice, replace the pepper jack cheese with mozzarella.

• For a complete meal, feel free to toss some veggies, such as bell peppers or califlower, into the slow cooker alongside the chicken.

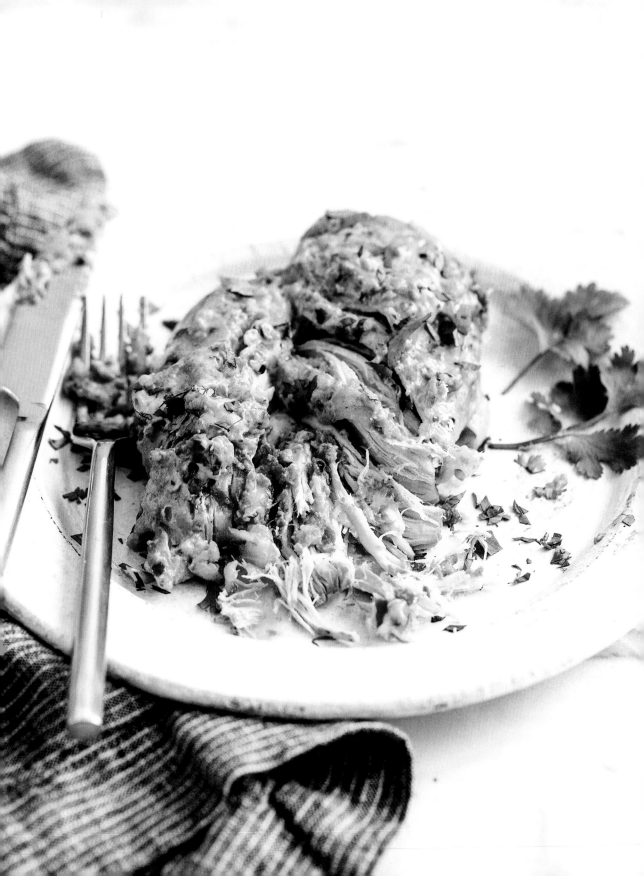

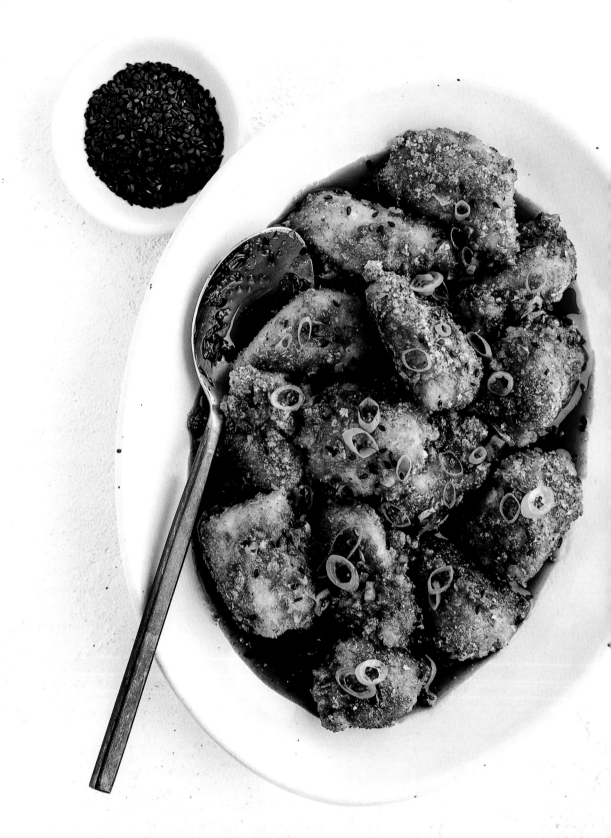

CRISPY ORANGE CHICKEN

There are hidden carbs lurking in most Chinese take-out dishes. Skipping the rice is not enough—you also have to watch for starchy breading, flour used to thicken sauces, and sugar. This recipe adapts one of the most popular Chinese meals, orange chicken, to be keto-friendly, with no need for any starches or sugar. You might not even notice that there is a difference!

1. **Prepare the chicken:** Season the chicken with sea salt and black pepper.

2. In a small bowl, whisk the eggs. In a medium bowl, place the crushed pork rinds.

3. In a large skillet, heat the oil over medium-high heat.

4. Dip the chicken pieces in the egg, shake off the excess, then coat with the pork rind crumbs on all sides. (Alternatively, you can place all the chicken pieces in the egg at once, and take them out one by one to dip in the crumbs.) Working in batches, place a single layer of chicken into the pan. Cook for a few minutes on each side, until golden and cooked through.

5. Remove the chicken from the pan and cover with foil to keep warm. Repeat with the remaining chicken pieces. Keep the skillet for the sauce.

6. **Make the orange sauce:** While the chicken rests, in the same skillet, heat the oil over medium heat. Add the garlic and sauté for about 1 minute, until fragrant.

7. Add the coconut aminos, wine vinegar, orange zest, powdered erythritol, and ground ginger. Use a wooden spoon to scrape any browned bits from the bottom and deglaze the pan.

CHICKEN

- 1 *pound* boneless, skinless chicken breast, cut into 1-inch pieces
- ½ *teaspoon* sea salt
- ¼ *teaspoon* black pepper
- 2 *large* eggs
- 3 *ounces* pork rinds, crushed to the texture of breadcrumbs
- 2 *tablespoons* avocado oil

ORANGE SAUCE

- 1 *tablespoon* avocado oil
- 2 *cloves* garlic, minced
- ½ *cup* coconut aminos
- ¼ *cup* white wine vinegar
- 2 *tablespoons* orange zest
- 2 *tablespoons* (0.6 ounce) powdered erythritol
- ½ *teaspoon* ground ginger

MAKES 4 SERVINGS

SERVING SIZE
1 cup, about 6 chicken pieces (6 ounces)

PER SERVING
328 calories
18 g fat
12 g total carbs
7 g net carbs
29 g protein

recipe continues . . .

MEAT & FISH ENTRÉES

8. Bring the sauce to a gentle boil, reduce the heat, and simmer for 8 to 10 minutes, until the volume is reduced, and the sauce thickens and looks glossy.

9. Return the chicken to the pan and toss to coat. The sauce will thicken as it cools from hot to warm.

TIPS & VARIATIONS • If you have any trouble getting the pork rind crumbs to stick, you can dust the chicken lightly with coconut flour before dipping it into the egg wash.

• If you are not grain-free, you can use rice vinegar instead of white wine vinegar. This is more common in Chinese cooking.

• The easiest way to make crushed pork rinds is in a blender or food processor. Alternatively, for less cleanup, you can place the pork rinds into a large bag and pound with the flat side of a meat mallet.

• This recipe makes a mild orange chicken. If you like some heat, add a sprinkle of red pepper flakes to the sauce: ⅛ to ¼ teaspoon, to taste. Green onions can also be used for garnish.

PAN-SEARED STEAK WITH MUSHROOM SAUCE

If you think you need to go to a fancy steakhouse to have a great steak, think again! It's actually super simple to make perfect steak at home, and doesn't take very long at all. The key is searing a piece of high-quality meat over high heat, followed by a few minutes in the oven, then letting it rest at the end. This recipe combines a classic sirloin with a rich, creamy mushroom sauce.

1. Season the steaks on both sides with the sea salt and black pepper. Let rest at room temperature for 30 minutes.

2. Heat a large sauté pan over medium-high heat. Add 2 tablespoons of the butter and melt.

3. Place the steaks in the pan in a single layer. Cook for the following number of minutes on each side, based on desired level of doneness (cook time will vary depending on the steak's thickness and the temperature of the pan). For best results, use a meat thermometer and remove the steak from the heat when it's 5°F lower than the desired final temperature. Steaks will rise another 5°F while resting.

Rare: 2 to 4 minutes per side, or until 115°F inside.
Steak will reach 120°F while resting afterward.

Medium-rare: 3 to 5 minutes per side, or until 125°F inside.
Steak will reach 130°F while resting afterward.

Medium: 4 to 6 minutes per side, or until 135°F inside.
Steak will reach 140°F while resting afterward.

Medium-well: 5 to 7 minutes per side, or until 145°F inside.
Steak will reach 150°F while resting afterward.

Well-done: 7 to 9 minutes per side, or until 155°F inside.
Steak will reach 160°F while resting afterward.

4 top sirloin steaks (6 ounces each), at room temperature

½ teaspoon sea salt, or more to taste

¼ teaspoon black pepper, or more to taste

4 tablespoons (½ stick) butter, divided into 2 tablespoons and 2 tablespoons

2 cloves garlic, minced

8 ounces (~3 cups) baby portobello mushrooms, thinly sliced

¼ cup beef broth

1 teaspoon fresh thyme, chopped

¼ cup heavy cream

MAKES 4 SERVINGS

SERVING SIZE
1 steak (4.5 ounces) with ¼ cup mushroom sauce

PER SERVING
420 calories
27 g fat
3 g total carbs
3 g net carbs
39 g protein

recipe continues . . .

MEAT & FISH ENTRÉES

4. When the steaks in the pan reach the desired internal temperature, remove them from the pan, transfer to a plate, and cover with foil. Let the steaks rest without cutting: the steak's internal temperature will rise another 5°F to the desired final temperature.

5. Return the sauté pan to medium heat. Melt the remaining 2 tablespoons butter. Add the garlic and sauté for about 1 minute, until fragrant.

6. Add the mushrooms, beef broth, and thyme. Scrape any browned bits from the bottom of the pan. Adjust the heat to bring to a simmer (typically at medium-high), cover, and simmer, stirring occasionally, for 5 to 8 minutes, until the mushrooms are soft.

7. Reduce the heat to medium, add the cream, and simmer for 1 to 3 minutes, until the sauce thickens. Adjust salt and pepper to taste, if needed.

8. Spoon the mushroom sauce over the steaks to serve.

TIPS & VARIATIONS • Do not cut or pierce the steak with a knife to see if it's done—this will release the juices and make it dry. A meat thermometer is a better method to check for doneness.

• Be careful not to overcook the mushroom sauce or get the heat too high, because either of these can cause it to separate.

• For a dairy-free version, use coconut oil instead of butter and coconut cream instead of heavy cream.

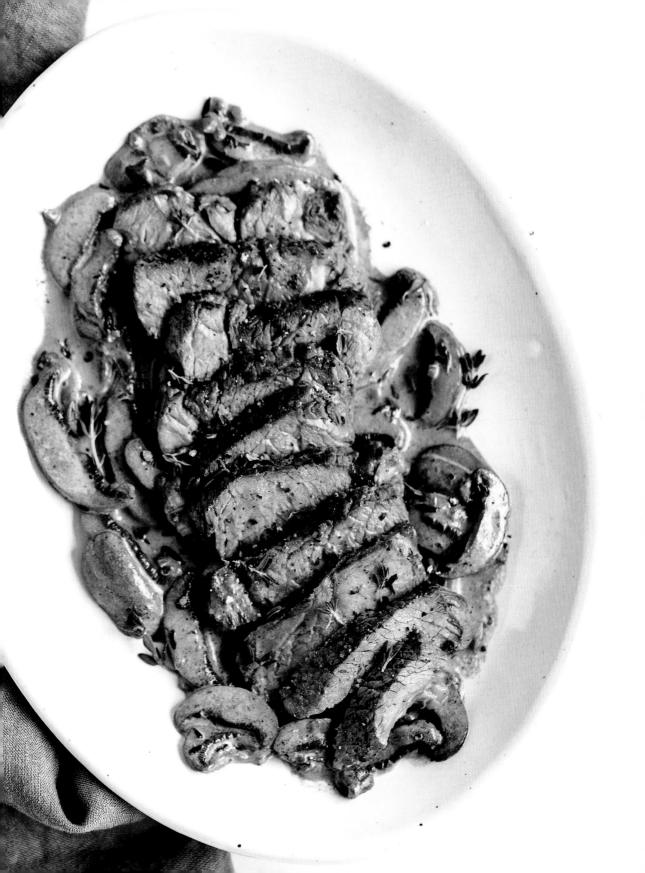

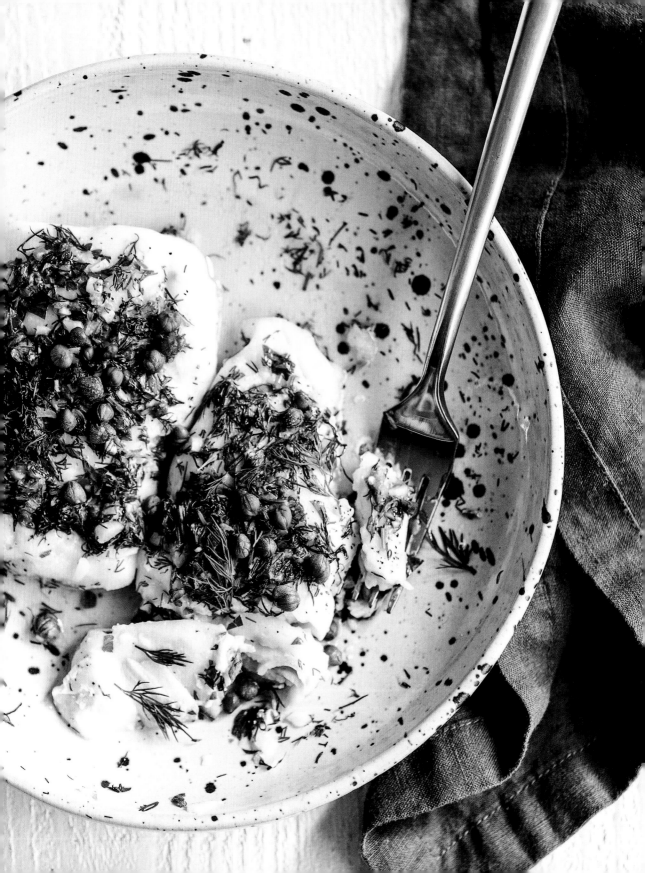

SIMPLE LEMON-HERB WHITEFISH

The term "whitefish" actually encompasses at least half a dozen different species of fish, but the "real" one is lake whitefish, found in the Great Lakes. If you can get it, it's one of the best to use for this keto recipe due to its higher fat content and mild flavor. However, many other types of fish will also work—check the tips for recommended alternatives.

1. Preheat the oven to 400°F. Line a sheet pan with foil or parchment paper and grease lightly.

2. Place the fish fillets in a single layer on the pan. Season the fish on both sides with the sea salt and black pepper.

3. In a small bowl, whisk together the oil, lemon zest, lemon juice, garlic, capers (if using), parsley, and dill. Spoon about 1 tablespoon of the lemon-herb oil over each piece of fish, then use a brush to spread it.

4. Bake for 10 to 14 minutes, depending on the thickness of the fish, until the fish flakes easily with a fork.

TIPS & VARIATIONS · If you can't locate lake whitefish, you can use other fatty white fish species, such as halibut or grouper. Leaner types of fish, like tilapia, cod, or flounder, also work if you can balance the meal with a higher-fat side dish.

· If you are not dairy-free, try sprinkling some Parmesan cheese over the fish before baking.

· The herb topping has a bit of a gremolata flair with the capers. The recipe also works well without them, so you can leave them out if you're not a fan.

6 white fish fillets (~5 ounces each), preferably lake whitefish, grouper, or halibut

1 teaspoon sea salt

½ teaspoon black pepper

3 tablespoons olive oil

2 teaspoons lemon zest

2 teaspoons lemon juice

2 cloves garlic, minced

1 teaspoon minced capers (optional)

3 tablespoons minced fresh parsley

3 tablespoons minced fresh dill

MAKES 6 SERVINGS

SERVING SIZE
1 fillet (~4 ounces)

PER SERVING
325 calories
17 g fat
0 g total carbs
0 g net carbs
37 g protein

MEAT & FISH ENTREES

CHILI-LIME TURKEY BURGERS

Those of us who usually prefer beef tend to think that turkey burgers are dry or flavorless. It doesn't have to be that way—adding mayonnaise and zesty spices makes these chili-lime turkey burgers anything but! They are super juicy and fantastic for Mexican night.

1. In a large bowl, combine all the ingredients except the avocado oil. Use your hands to mix, being careful not to overmix.

2. Divide the meat into 4 portions and form into patties, ⅓ to ½ inch thick. Make a thumbprint in each.

3. In a sauté pan, heat the oil over medium to medium-high heat. Cook the burgers for 4 to 5 minutes per side, until cooked through.

TIPS & VARIATIONS • For best results, do not let the raw turkey meat sit at room temperature for any amount of time, which can lead to tough burgers. For the same reason, do not overmix the meat.

• Serve turkey burgers with Simple Guacamole (page 248), Pantry Staple Salsa (page 240), leaf lettuce, and Almond Flax Burger Buns (page 207).

• If you are not dairy-free, add a slice of cheese (pepper jack works well!) over the burgers at the end and cover with a lid to melt.

1 **pound** ground turkey

3 **tablespoons** 2-Minute Avocado Oil Mayonnaise (page 235)

1 **teaspoon** lime zest

1 **teaspoon** lime juice

1 **tablespoon** chili powder

¾ **teaspoon** sea salt

½ **teaspoon** dried oregano

¼ **teaspoon** garlic powder

⅛ **teaspoon** cayenne pepper (optional)

1 **tablespoon** avocado oil

MAKES 4 SERVINGS

SERVING SIZE

1 turkey burger (~3.5 ounces)

PER SERVING

283 calories

21 g fat

1 g total carbs

1 g net carbs

21 g protein

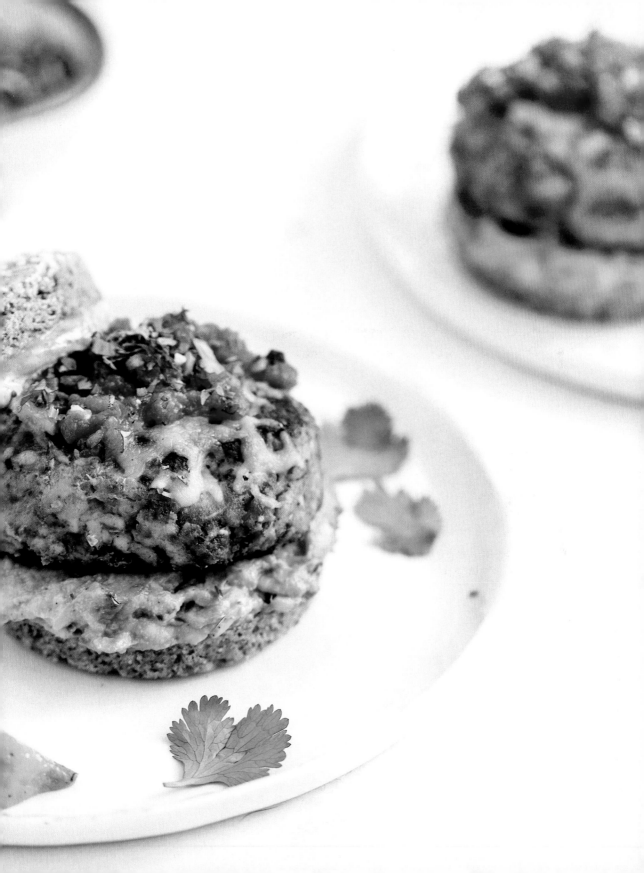

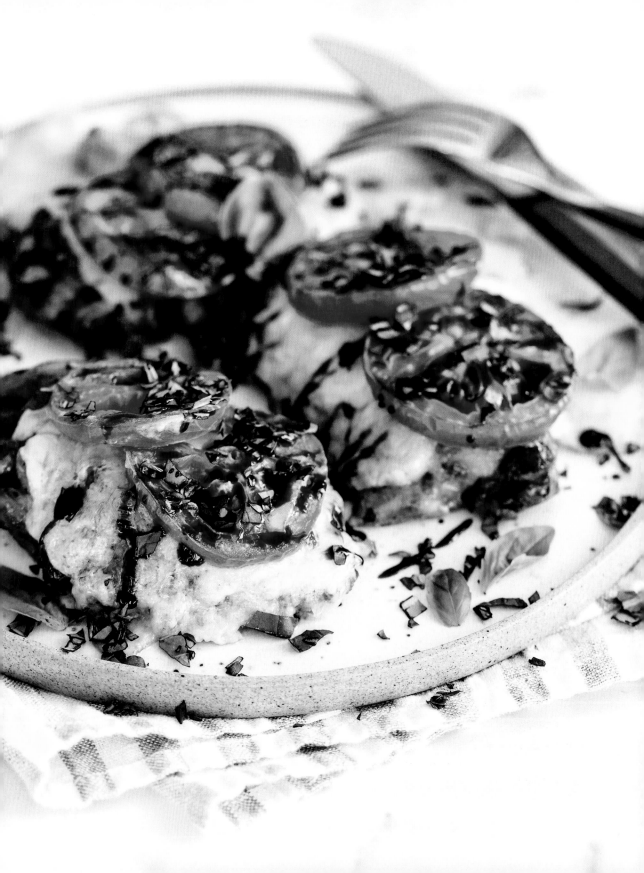

CAPRESE CHICKEN THIGHS

When we visited Italy a few years ago, I couldn't get enough of the Caprese salads. I brought that obsession back home with me, inspired to make Caprese anything and everything. These Caprese chicken thighs take all of those flavors and turn them into a satisfying main dish!

1. In a large bowl, whisk together the oil, 2 tablespoons of balsamic vinegar, the Italian seasoning, garlic powder, sea salt, and black pepper.

2. Add the chicken thighs and push down into the marinade. Set aside for 20 minutes, or refrigerate until ready to use.

3. Meanwhile, preheat the oven to 375°F. Line a sheet pan with foil or parchment paper.

4. Shake off any excess marinade from each piece of chicken and arrange on the baking sheet in a single layer without touching.

5. Top each chicken thigh with a slice of mozzarella, covering most of it. You may need to cut a piece in half to cover the chicken better. Place 2 slices of tomato on top of the mozzarella.

6. Roast for 23 to 28 minutes, until the chicken is cooked through. You may need to pour off extra liquid from the pan at the end.

7. Drizzle the chicken with the remaining 1 tablespoon balsamic vinegar (or with a reduction by simmering more balsamic vinegar in a small saucepan). Garnish with basil ribbons.

⅓ cup olive oil

3 tablespoons balsamic vinegar, divided into 2 tablespoons and 1 tablespoon

1 teaspoon Italian seasoning

½ teaspoon garlic powder

½ teaspoon sea salt

¼ teaspoon black pepper

8 boneless, skinless chicken thighs (~2.5 ounces each)

4 ounces fresh mozzarella cheese, cut into 8 slices (0.5 ounce each)

2 medium Roma (plum) tomatoes, thinly sliced

2 tablespoons fresh basil, cut into ribbons

MAKES 4 SERVINGS

SERVING SIZE
2 chicken thighs
(~5 ounces total)

PER SERVING
564 calories
46 g fat
4 g total carbs
4 g net carbs
31 g protein

TIPS & VARIATIONS • You can make the same recipe with chicken breasts if you'd like. Baking time will be reduced to 16 to 22 minutes, depending on the size of the breasts.

• This recipe is easy to prep ahead. You can marinate the chicken ahead of time and portion out the tomatoes, mozzarella, and basil until ready to assemble. Alternatively, you can even fully bake the chicken and then reheat.

MEAT & FISH ENTRÉES

KUNG PAO BEEF

I wasn't a huge fan of Chinese food growing up, mainly because I've never loved the white rice that comes with virtually every Chinese dish. In adulthood, I've grown to love this cuisine. I can easily skip the rice, but, ironically, now I've become a huge fan of cauliflower rice! Chinese meals, like this kung pao beef, have become one of my favorite types of recipes to adapt for the keto lifestyle. Whether you serve this stir-fry on its own or over cauliflower rice, it tastes just like take-out kung pao beef.

1. **Make the sauce/marinade:** In a small bowl, whisk together the coconut aminos, white wine vinegar, sherry wine, avocado oil, and chili paste.

2. **Make the stir-fry:** Place the sliced steak into a medium bowl. Pour half of the sauce/marinade (about ¼ cup) over it and stir to coat. Cover and chill for at least 30 minutes, up to 2 hours.

3. About 10 minutes before marinating time is up or when you are ready to cook, in a large wok or sauté pan, heat 1 tablespoon of the oil over medium-high heat. Add the bell peppers and sauté for 7 to 8 minutes, until soft and browned.

4. Add the garlic and sauté for about 1 minute, until fragrant.

5. Remove the peppers and garlic, and cover to keep warm.

6. Add the remaining 1 tablespoon oil to the pan and heat over very high heat. Add the steak, arrange in a single layer, and cook undisturbed for 2 to 4 minutes per side, until browned on each side. If it's not cooked through yet, you can stir-fry for longer. Remove the meat from the pan and cover to keep warm.

7. Add the reserved marinade to the pan. Bring to a vigorous simmer and continue to simmer for a few minutes, until thickened.

8. Add the cooked meat, cooked peppers, and roasted peanuts to the pan and toss in the sauce.

SAUCE/MARINADE

- ¼ *cup* coconut aminos
- 1½ *tablespoons* white wine vinegar
- 1½ *tablespoons* sherry wine
- 1 *tablespoon* avocado oil
- 1 *teaspoon* chili paste

STIR-FRY

- 1 *pound* flank steak, thinly sliced against the grain and cut into bite-size pieces
- 2 *tablespoons* avocado oil, divided into 1 tablespoon and 1 tablespoon
- 2 *medium* bell peppers (6 ounces each), red and green, chopped into bite-size pieces
- 2 *cloves* garlic, minced
- ¼ *cup* roasted peanuts

MAKES 4 SERVINGS

SERVING SIZE
1 cup (6 ounces)

PER SERVING
341 calories
20 g fat
9 g total carbs
7 g net carbs
27 g protein

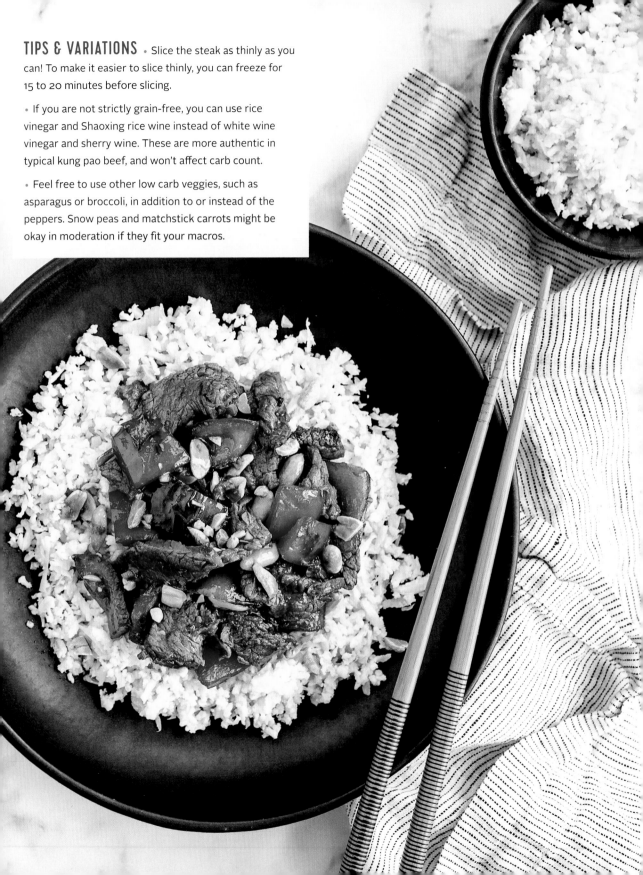

TIPS & VARIATIONS • Slice the steak as thinly as you can! To make it easier to slice thinly, you can freeze for 15 to 20 minutes before slicing.

• If you are not strictly grain-free, you can use rice vinegar and Shaoxing rice wine instead of white wine vinegar and sherry wine. These are more authentic in typical kung pao beef, and won't affect carb count.

• Feel free to use other low carb veggies, such as asparagus or broccoli, in addition to or instead of the peppers. Snow peas and matchstick carrots might be okay in moderation if they fit your macros.

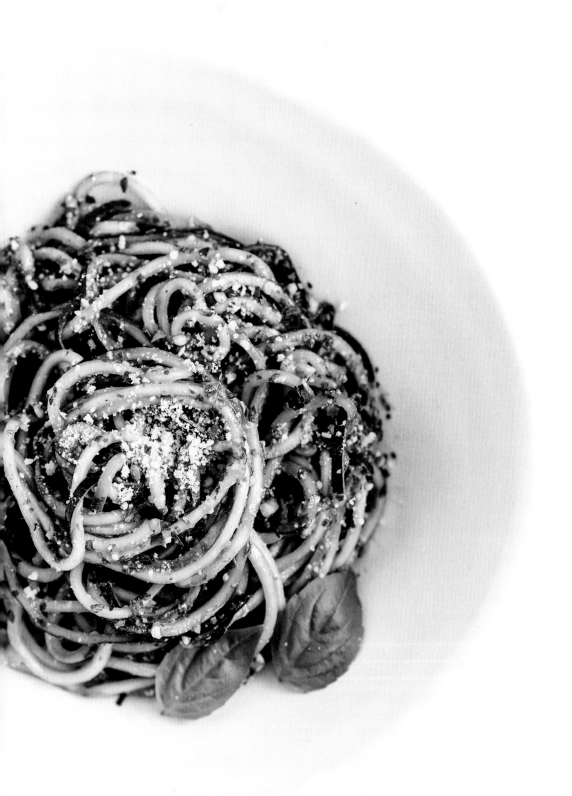

VEGGIES & SIDE DISHES

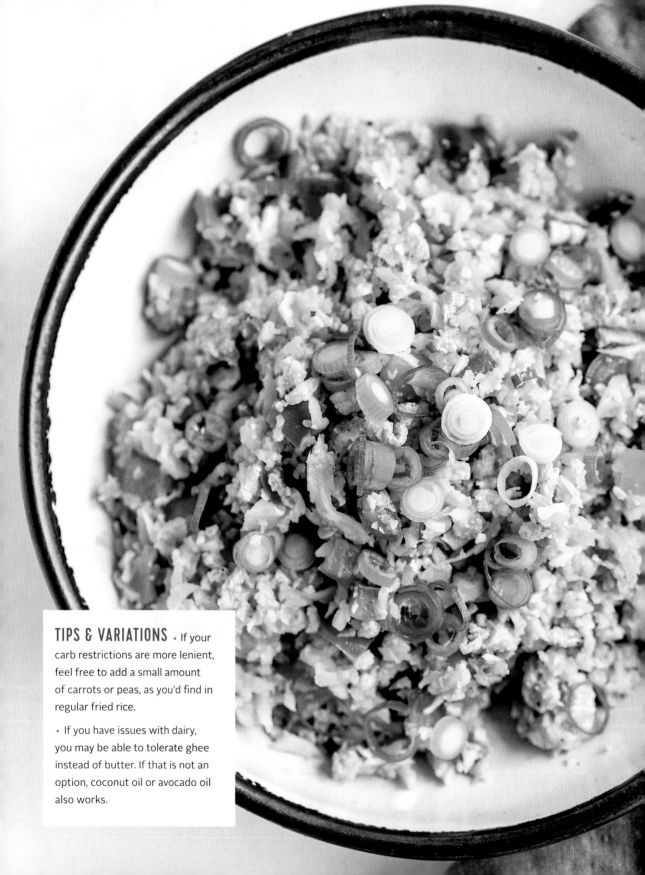

TIPS & VARIATIONS • If your carb restrictions are more lenient, feel free to add a small amount of carrots or peas, as you'd find in regular fried rice.

• If you have issues with dairy, you may be able to tolerate ghee instead of butter. If that is not an option, coconut oil or avocado oil also works.

CAULIFLOWER FRIED RICE

Traditional fried rice is usually made with carrots and peas, but both are fairly high in carbs and should only be enjoyed in moderation on the keto diet. Some people prefer to avoid them altogether, so in this recipe we replace them with bell peppers in the same bright colors! You'll still get all the flavor you'd expect from fried rice with a fraction of the carbs.

1. Remove the cauliflower leaves and stems. (Cut off as much of the stems as you can.) Push the cauliflower florets into a running food processor with a grating attachment, to make cauliflower rice. Alternatively, rice the cauliflower using a box grater.

2. In a large sauté pan, heat 1 tablespoon of the butter over medium heat. Add the bell peppers and sauté for about 5 minutes, until the peppers are soft. Add the garlic and sauté for about 1 minute, until fragrant.

3. Meanwhile, whisk the eggs with ¼ teaspoon sea salt and a pinch of black pepper.

4. Push the veggies to one side of the skillet. (If the pan is dry, you can melt in more butter.) Add the whisked eggs to the other side and cook for a few minutes, until barely scrambled.

5. Push everything to the side again and add the remaining 1 tablespoon butter to the pan. Once it melts, increase the heat to medium-high, immediately add the cauliflower rice, and stir everything together. Season with 1 teaspoon sea salt and ¼ teaspoon black pepper, or to taste. Stir-fry for about 5 minutes, until the cauliflower is soft but not mushy.

6. Remove from the heat. Stir in the coconut aminos, sesame oil, and green onions.

1 *head* cauliflower (to yield 2 pounds or 4 cups riced cauliflower)

2 *tablespoons* butter, divided into 1 tablespoon and 1 tablespoon

½ *medium* orange bell pepper (3 ounces), finely diced

½ *medium* green bell pepper (3 ounces), finely diced

3 *cloves* garlic, minced

2 *large* eggs

1¼ *teaspoon* sea salt, divided into ¼ teaspoon and 1 teaspoon

¼ *teaspoon* black pepper

2 *tablespoons* coconut aminos

1 *teaspoon* toasted sesame oil

3 green onions, chopped

MAKES 6 CUPS (6 SERVINGS)

SERVING SIZE
1 cup (~5 ounces)

PER SERVING
106 calories
6 g fat
8 g total carbs
6 g net carbs
4 g protein

VEGGIES & SIDE DISHES

GARLIC-HERB ROASTED RADISHES

When you're looking for a potato replacement for the keto lifestyle, think about less starchy vegetables that you can use in similar preparations. Radishes certainly fit the bill! These garlic-herb roasted radishes are reminiscent of skin-on baby red potatoes, and they pair beautifully with chicken or steak.

1. Preheat the oven to 425°F. Line a baking sheet with foil and grease it.

2. In a large bowl, whisk together the oil, garlic, thyme, rosemary, sea salt, and black pepper. Add the radishes and toss to coat.

3. Arrange the radishes in a single layer on the pan, making sure each one touches the pan. Spread them out as much as possible. Roast for 8 to 13 minutes, until golden on the bottom. Flip and roast for 8 to 13 more minutes.

TIPS & VARIATIONS • Baking time might vary depending on the size of your radishes. Check on them and flip when they start to get golden on the bottom.

• Foil is recommended over parchment paper to ensure good browning.

• Avocado oil is used because it has a higher smoke point than other cooking oils. If you like a buttery flavor, you can toss the radishes with a bit of melted butter after roasting.

3 tablespoons avocado oil

3 cloves garlic, minced

1 tablespoon fresh thyme, chopped

1 tablespoon fresh rosemary, chopped

1½ teaspoons sea salt

¼ teaspoon black pepper

2 pounds (~40) radishes, trimmed and halved

MAKES 3 CUPS (6 SERVINGS)

SERVING SIZE
½ cup (~3 ounces)

PER SERVING
98 calories
7 g fat
6 g total carbs
4 g net carbs
1 g protein

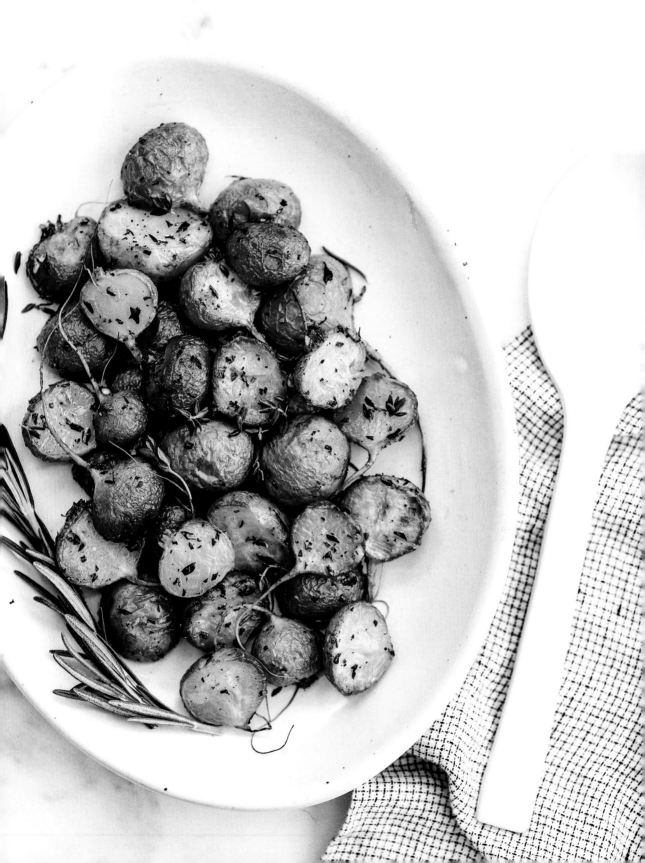

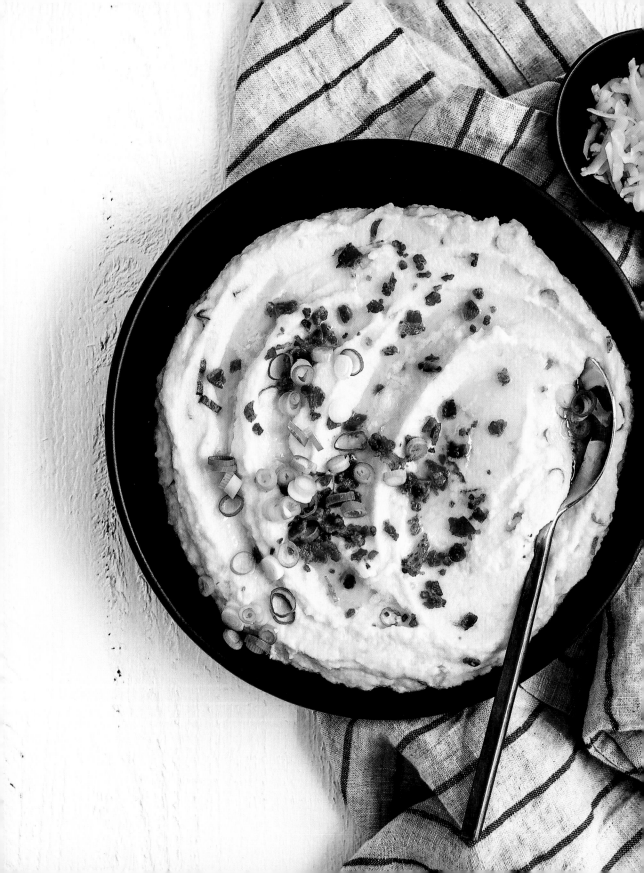

LOADED CAULIFLOWER MASH

Cauliflower mash is the most common keto substitute for mashed potatoes. You may be skeptical if you're not a huge fan of cauliflower, but I encourage you to try out this recipe—you'll be amazed by how much this mash tastes like the real thing! Loaded cauliflower mash has all the same flavors as regular loaded mashed potatoes. The cauliflower flavor takes a back seat to the ultrarich butter, cream, cheese, and bacon.

1. Bring a large pot of water to a boil on the stove top. Add the cauliflower florets and cook for 8 to 10 minutes, until very soft. Drain well and pat dry.

2. Meanwhile, in a microwave-safe bowl or in a saucepan, combine the butter, sour cream, heavy cream, garlic, and sea salt, and heat in the microwave or on the stove until hot and melted.

3. Transfer the cauliflower florets to a food processor. Add the butter-cream mixture and puree until smooth.

4. Transfer the cauliflower to a serving dish. Immediately stir in most of the cheddar, bacon bits, and green onions, reserving a little of each for the topping. To serve, garnish with the reserved cheddar, bacon, and green onions.

TIPS & VARIATIONS

• Unlike the typical method of blanching cauliflower, in this recipe you don't need an ice water bath. Since we are pureeing the cauliflower, it doesn't matter if it overcooks or gets too soft. And when you're making a mash, the softer, the better! It should be almost mashing together when you drain it.

• The total recipe yield will vary slightly depending on the size of your cauliflower—you may get more or less mash. The serving *size* remains the same, but the nutrition info may vary slightly depending on how many servings you get.

• The hot cauliflower should melt the cheddar if you stir it in right away. If it doesn't, you can place the mashed cauliflower under the broiler for a few minutes to melt it.

---

1 *head* cauliflower, cut into florets (~4 cups or 2 pounds florets)

2 *tablespoons* butter

¼ *cup* sour cream

2 *tablespoons* heavy cream

3 *cloves* garlic, minced

1 *teaspoon* sea salt

1½ *cups (6 ounces)* shredded cheddar cheese

⅓ *cup* cooked bacon bits

¼ *cup (0.9 ounce)* chopped green onions

MAKES 4 CUPS (8 SERVINGS)

SERVING SIZE
½ cup (~4 ounces)

PER SERVING
180 calories
13 g fat
5 g total carbs
3 g net carbs
9 g protein

VEGGIES & SIDE DISHES

FATHEAD GNOCCHI

I tried making fathead gnocchi on a whim. I was pleasantly surprised to find that it worked! These soft pillows of pure comfort used to be one of my favorite carb-filled side dishes, so re-creating them was pretty exciting. Fathead dough makes wonderful keto gnocchi, as long as you don't boil them. (Don't—they will disintegrate!) And that's just as well, because the crispy sautéed version or soft golden baked versions are even more delicious. They are incredibly filling, too!

1. Make the fathead dough through Step 2 of the instructions on pages 17 to 19. If it's too sticky to work with, refrigerate for 30 minutes.

2. Use a small cookie scoop (2-teaspoon size) to pick up a small ball of dough. Tear in half and shape or roll to make two gnocchi from each scoop. (Alternatively, you can just use a teaspoon for each gnocchi right away, but I find that splitting the 2-teaspoon cookie scoop makes it easier to portion them out.) If desired, roll the gnocchi over the back of a fork to make the typical gnocchi ridges.

3. In a sauté pan, heat 2 tablespoons of the oil over medium-low to medium heat. Add the gnocchi in a single layer. Sauté for 3 to 5 minutes, until golden on the bottom. Flip and sauté for 3 to 5 more minutes, until golden on the bottom and cooked through. They burn easily if the heat is too high, so adjust as needed based on your stove.

4. Toss the gnocchi with the remaining 1 tablespoon oil, Parmesan, and parsley. Sprinkle each serving with a little extra Parmesan, if desired.

1 *recipe* Fathead Dough (page 17), made with baking powder

3 *tablespoons* olive oil, divided into 2 tablespoons and 1 tablespoon

3 *tablespoons (0.75 ounce)* grated Parmesan cheese, plus more for garnish

½ *tablespoon* chopped fresh parsley

MAKES 2 CUPS (4 SERVINGS)

SERVING SIZE
½ cup, or 9 to 12 gnocchi (2.5 ounces)

PER SERVING
ALMOND FLOUR VERSION
398 calories
35 g fat
6 g total carbs
4 g net carbs
16 g protein

COCONUT FLOUR VERSION
344 calories
27 g fat
7 g total carbs
4 g net carbs
15 g protein

TIPS & VARIATIONS • The sauté method makes a golden, crispy exterior, which I prefer. For a lighter option, you can bake them in the oven for 10 minutes at 375°F instead.

• Watch the gnocchi closely when pan-frying—they burn easily. Low heat makes lightly golden gnocchi, medium-low makes them darker golden.

• You can form the gnocchi ahead of time, place them on a pan lined with parchment paper, and refrigerate or freeze. Pan-fry right before serving.

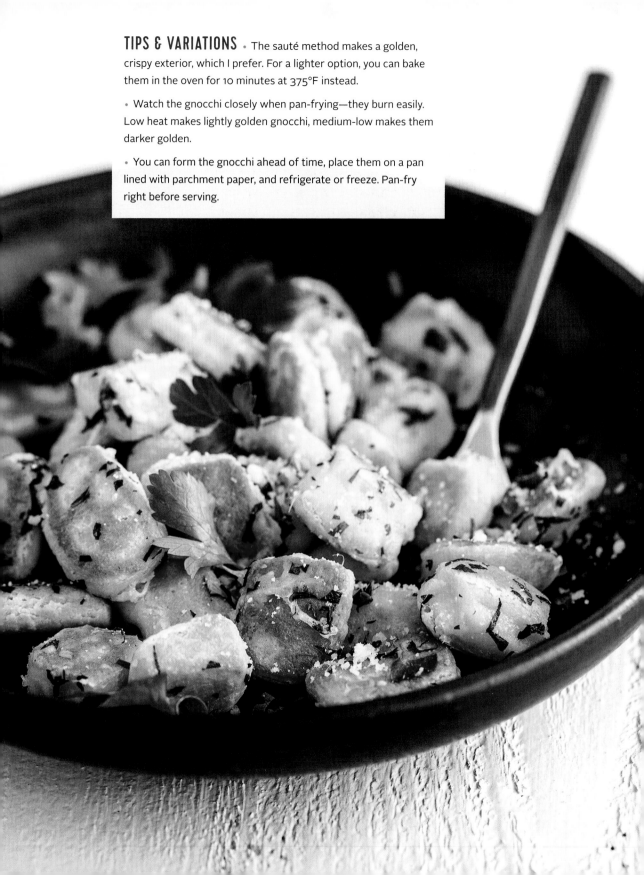

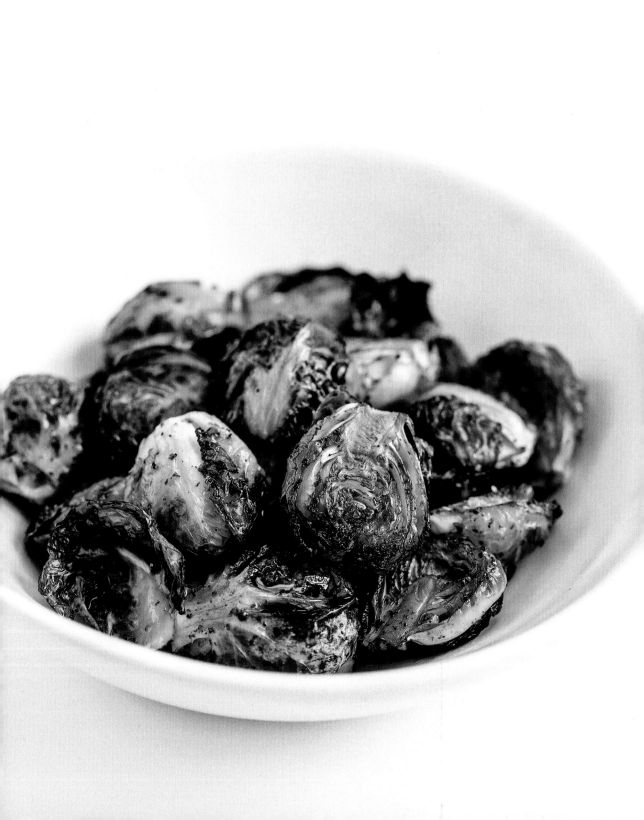

BALSAMIC ROASTED BRUSSELS SPROUTS

If the thought of Brussels sprouts makes you cringe, it's time to try a new method. Roasting them at a high temperature makes for beautifully browned and crispy sprouts that taste indulgent. And even if you roast Brussels sprouts all the time, it's amazing how much a splash of balsamic vinegar enhances the flavor!

¼ *cup* olive oil

2 *tablespoons* balsamic vinegar

½ *teaspoon* garlic powder

1 *teaspoon* sea salt

¼ *teaspoon* black pepper

1 *pound (~24)* Brussels sprouts, trimmed and halved

MAKES 4 CUPS (8 SERVINGS)

SERVING SIZE
½ cup (~2 ounces)

PER SERVING
88 calories
6 g fat
5 g total carbs
3 g net carbs
1 g protein

1. Preheat the oven to 450°F. Line a large baking sheet with foil.

2. In a large bowl, whisk together the oil, balsamic vinegar, garlic powder, sea salt, and black pepper, until smooth. Add the Brussels sprouts and toss to coat.

3. Spread the Brussels sprouts over the baking sheet in a single layer, so that all the sprouts touch the pan. Roast for 10 to 15 minutes, until browned on the bottom. Flip and repeat for another 10 to 15 minutes.

TIPS & VARIATIONS • For extra flavor, you can replace some of the olive oil with bacon grease. You can also toss the Brussels sprouts with bacon bits at the end.

• For best results, use an extra-large pan and spread the Brussels sprouts in a single layer. This improves airflow around the sprouts, ensuring crispier edges.

LEMON-GARLIC ROASTED BROCCOLI

I'm all about easy side dishes, and this roasted broccoli is one of my favorites with the simple twist of lemon juice and zest for flavor. Roasting at the perfect temperature of 400°F creates beautifully browned, crispy florets—the best kind, right?

1. Preheat the oven to 400°F. Grease a 20 × 14-inch baking sheet or two 10 × 14-inch pans.

2. In a large bowl, whisk together the oil, lemon zest, lemon juice, garlic, sea salt, and black pepper. (You can tilt the bowl to the side to help when whisking this small amount in a large bowl.)

3. Add the broccoli florets and toss to coat.

4. Arrange the broccoli florets in a single layer on the baking sheet so that each piece is touching the baking sheet.

5. Roast for 20 to 30 minutes, until the edges of the florets are browned.

TIPS & VARIATIONS • If you don't have fresh garlic, you can use minced garlic from a jar (1 teaspoon = 1 clove) or garlic powder (½ teaspoon = 1 clove).

• This recipe also works with cauliflower, or a blend of broccoli and cauliflower.

• Feel free to add other spices, like paprika or Italian seasoning.

¼ *cup* olive oil

1 *teaspoon* lemon zest

1 *tablespoon* lemon juice

6 *cloves* garlic, minced

½ *teaspoon* sea salt

¼ *teaspoon* black pepper

1 *pound (~8 cups)* broccoli florets

MAKES 6 SERVINGS

SERVING SIZE
1 cup (~2 ounces)

PER SERVING
109 calories
9 g fat
5 g total carbs
3 g net carbs
2 g protein

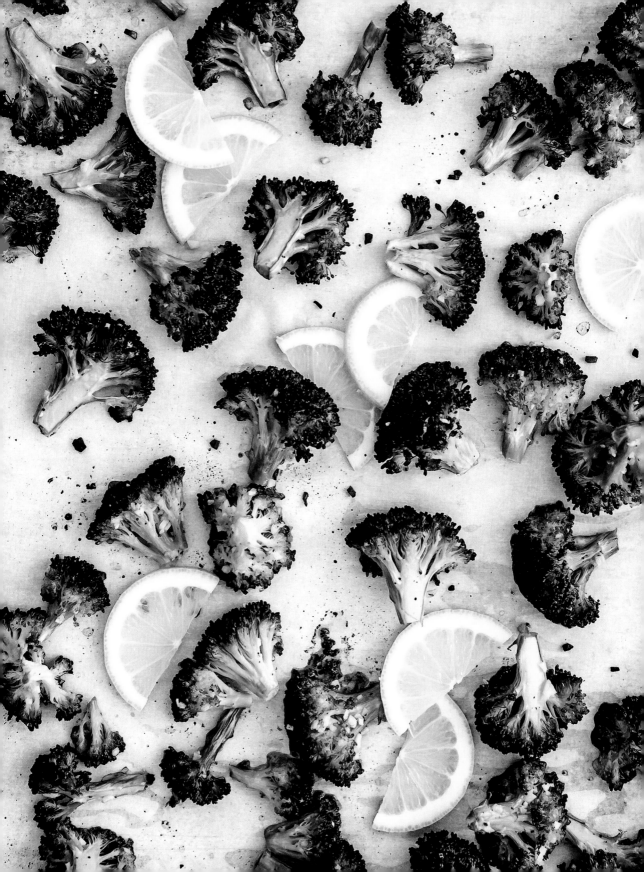

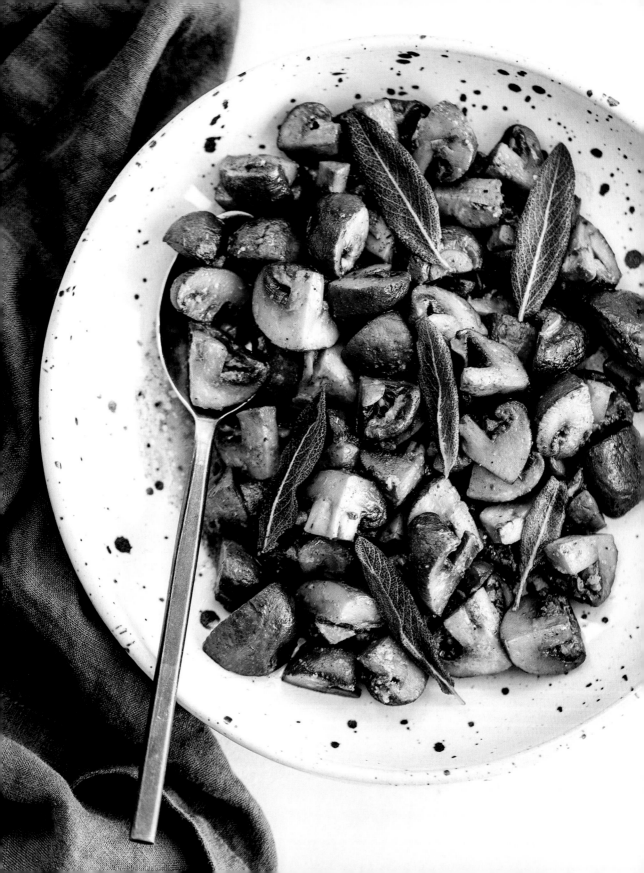

BROWNED BUTTER SAGE MUSHROOMS

Keto side dish options often revolve around green vegetables, so sautéed mushrooms are a nice change of pace. Made with browned butter and sage, a less commonly used herb, this side dish is anything but boring. And the cooking time is only about 15 minutes, so you can get it on the table fast!

5 *tablespoons* butter, divided into 4 tablespoons and 1 tablespoon

¼ *teaspoon* ground sage

2 *cloves* garlic, minced

1 *pound (~5 cups)* baby portobello mushrooms, cut into quarters

½ *teaspoon* sea salt

⅛ *teaspoon* black pepper

8 *medium* fresh sage leaves

MAKES 4 CUPS (8 SERVINGS)

1. In a large sauté pan, melt 4 tablespoons of the butter over medium heat. Add the dried sage and heat for 2 to 3 minutes, stirring occasionally, until the butter starts to turn golden.

2. Add the garlic and heat for another 2 to 3 minutes, until the butter is dark golden brown and smells nutty. Watch the pan closely, because the butter can go from browned to burned quickly.

3. Add the mushrooms. Sprinkle with sea salt and black pepper. Cover and cook for 7 to 10 minutes, lifting the lid to stir occasionally, until the mushrooms are soft and most of the moisture evaporates. Uncover and stir-fry for another couple minutes to evaporate any remaining excess moisture. Remove the mushrooms from the pan and cover to keep warm.

4. Melt the remaining 1 tablespoon butter in the pan. Add the fresh sage leaves in a single layer. Fry for just a few seconds, until crispy.

5. Use the crispy sage leaves for topping the mushrooms—whole for garnish or crumbled for flavor.

SERVING SIZE
½ cup (~2.5 ounces)

PER SERVING
154 calories
14 g fat
4 g total carbs
3 g net carbs
2 g protein

TIPS & VARIATIONS · The same recipe works with other herbs. Try adding some fresh thyme or rosemary. You'll need the same amount as sage if using dried herbs, or triple the amount for fresh herbs.

· Feel free to include a mix of mushrooms, like button, shiitake, or other wild mushrooms.

VEGGIES & SIDE DISHES

ALMOND PESTO ZUCCHINI NOODLES

Before I went low carb, one of my favorite meals used to be a big bowl of noodles with pesto sauce. I still like to re-create this in a keto-friendly way, by using zucchini noodles instead. This recipe makes homemade pesto using almonds, which are easier to find and cheaper than pine nuts. It has an excellent fat-to-protein ratio for a keto lifestyle, plus it's filling enough for a meatless meal.

1. In a colander set in the sink, toss the zucchini noodles with ¼ teaspoon of the sea salt. Let sit for 30 minutes to drain, then squeeze to release more water. You don't have to get every last drop out, just most of it. Pat dry.

2. Meanwhile, preheat the oven to 400°F.

3. Arrange the almonds in a single layer on a baking sheet. Toast in the oven for 6 to 8 minutes, until golden and fragrant. Watch them carefully so they don't burn.

4. Transfer the almonds to a food processor. Pulse a few times until the almonds are broken up into coarse pieces—don't overmix.

5. Add the basil, Parmesan, olive oil, garlic, pepper, and remaining ½ teaspoon sea salt. Pulse on and off, scraping the sides occasionally, until you get a pesto consistency. Adjust sea salt and black pepper to taste—it should be on the salty side, as this will be diluted when you add the zucchini noodles.

6. In a large sauté pan, heat the avocado oil over medium-high heat. Add the zucchini noodles and stir-fry for 3 to 4 minutes, until al dente.

7. Add the pesto and toss to coat. Stir-fry for just 1 more minute, until hot. Serve immediately.

4 *medium* zucchini (1¼ pounds total), spiralized

¾ *teaspoon* sea salt, divided into ¼ teaspoon and ½ teaspoon

⅓ *cup (1.7 ounces)* raw almonds

2 *packed cups (~4 ounces)* fresh basil

⅓ *cup (1.3 ounces)* grated Parmesan cheese

⅔ *cup* extra virgin olive oil

2 *cloves* garlic, cut into a few pieces

⅛ *teaspoon* black pepper

1 *tablespoon* avocado oil

MAKES 4 CUPS (4 SERVINGS)

SERVING SIZE
1 cup (5 ounces)

PER SERVING
492 calories
48 g fat
10 g total carbs
7 g net carbs
8 g protein

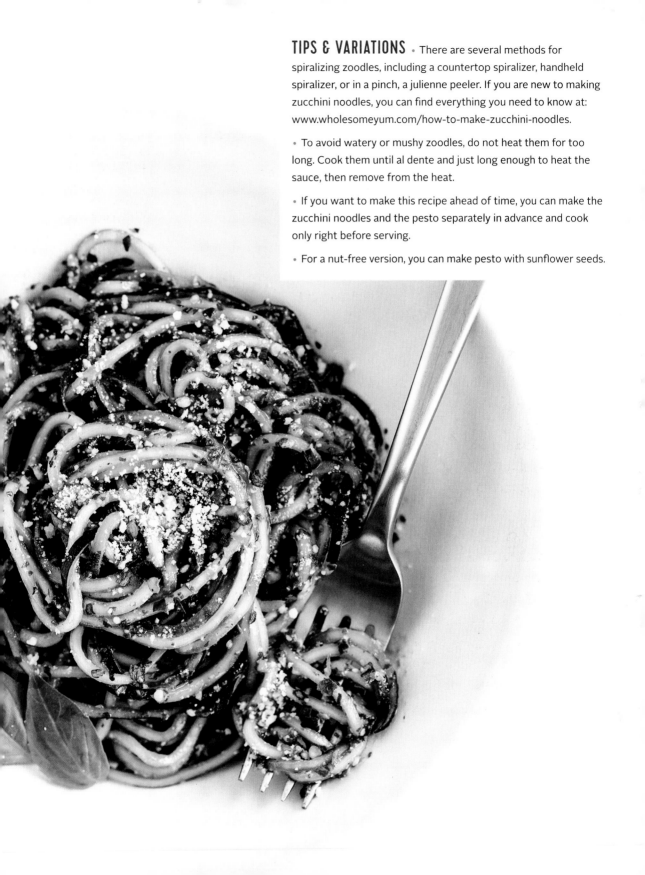

TIPS & VARIATIONS

· There are several methods for spiralizing zoodles, including a countertop spiralizer, handheld spiralizer, or in a pinch, a julienne peeler. If you are new to making zucchini noodles, you can find everything you need to know at: www.wholesomeyum.com/how-to-make-zucchini-noodles.

· To avoid watery or mushy zoodles, do not heat them for too long. Cook them until al dente and just long enough to heat the sauce, then remove from the heat.

· If you want to make this recipe ahead of time, you can make the zucchini noodles and the pesto separately in advance and cook only right before serving.

· For a nut-free version, you can make pesto with sunflower seeds.

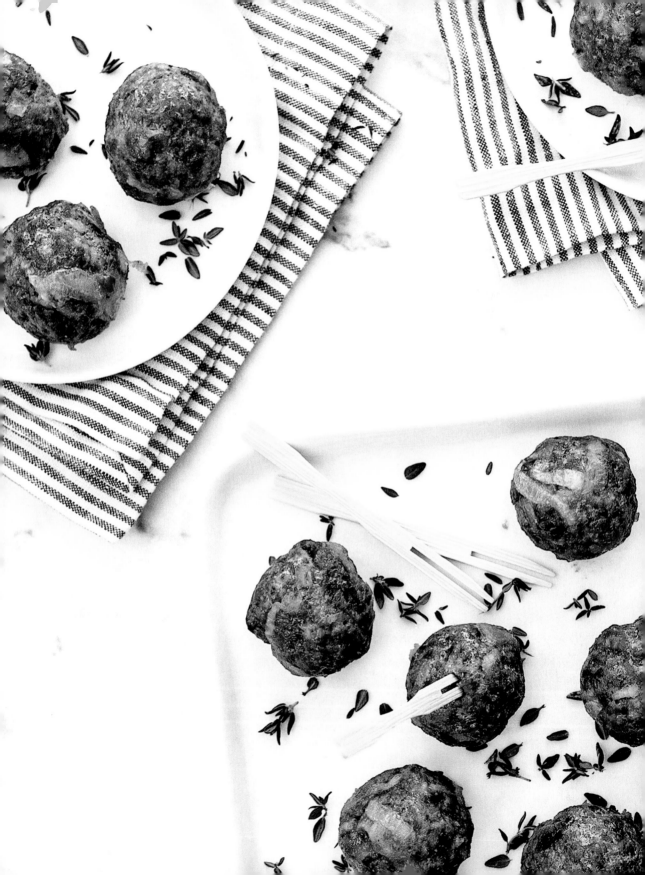

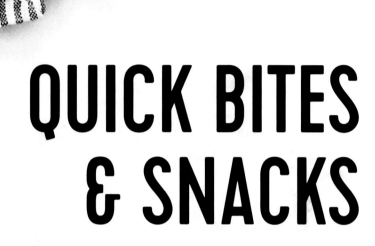

QUICK BITES & SNACKS

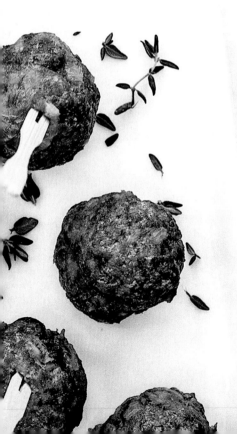

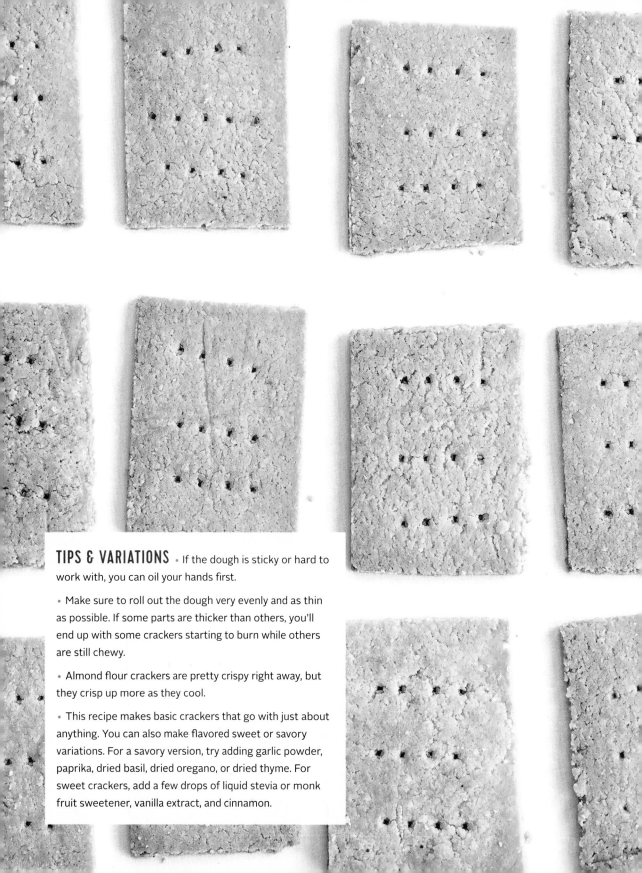

TIPS & VARIATIONS • If the dough is sticky or hard to work with, you can oil your hands first.

• Make sure to roll out the dough very evenly and as thin as possible. If some parts are thicker than others, you'll end up with some crackers starting to burn while others are still chewy.

• Almond flour crackers are pretty crispy right away, but they crisp up more as they cool.

• This recipe makes basic crackers that go with just about anything. You can also make flavored sweet or savory variations. For a savory version, try adding garlic powder, paprika, dried basil, dried oregano, or dried thyme. For sweet crackers, add a few drops of liquid stevia or monk fruit sweetener, vanilla extract, and cinnamon.

3-INGREDIENT ALMOND FLOUR CRACKERS

When you're missing the crunch of chips or crackers, almond flour crackers come to the rescue! It's pretty incredible how just three keto-friendly ingredients come together to make crackers that taste so much like their carb-packed counterparts from the grocery store! Eat these plain, or pair them with anything you'd normally put on crackers—cheese, nut butter, or creative toppings for mini party appetizers.

2 cups (8 ounces) blanched almond flour

½ teaspoon sea salt

1 large egg, beaten

MAKES 6 SERVINGS

SERVING SIZE
5 crackers (~1.3 ounces), or ⅙ of entire recipe

PER SERVING
226 calories
19 g fat
8 g total carbs
4 g net carbs
9 g protein

1. Preheat the oven to 350°F. Line a large baking sheet with parchment paper.

2. In a large bowl, mix together the almond flour and sea salt. Add the egg and mix well, until a dense, crumbly dough forms. (You can also mix in a food processor if you prefer.)

3. Place the dough between two large pieces of parchment paper. Use a rolling pin to roll out to a very thin rectangle, about ¹⁄₁₆ inch thick. (It will tend to roll into an oval shape, so just rip off pieces of dough and re-attach to form a more rectangular shape.)

4. Cut the cracker dough into rectangles. Place on the lined baking sheet. Prick with a fork a few times. Bake for 8 to 12 minutes, until golden.

QUICK BITES & SNACKS

EASY BAKED ZUCCHINI CHIPS

I'm always on the lookout for light, keto-friendly snacks that I can munch on without racking up too many carbs. Zucchini chips are a great option as they are light on carbs *and* calories, plus I love that I'm getting in an extra serving of veggies.

2 *medium* zucchini (10 ounces total)

1 *tablespoon* olive oil or avocado oil

½ *teaspoon* sea salt

MAKES 4 SERVINGS

SERVING SIZE
12 chips
(about ¼ cup/0.25 ounce)

PER SERVING
46 calories
4 g fat
4 g total carbs
2 g net carbs
2 g protein

1. Preheat the oven to 200°F.

2. Use a mandoline or a sharp knife to slice the zucchini into ⅛-inch-thick slices.

3. Place the zucchini in a large bowl. Add the olive oil and toss to thoroughly coat. Sprinkle lightly with sea salt. Toss to coat again.

4. Place ovenproof wire cooling racks on top of two baking sheets, then top those with parchment paper. (The cooling rack method allows for better air circulation.) Arrange the zucchini slices in a single layer. It's fine if they touch, but make sure they don't overlap.

5. Bake side by side for about 2½ hours, rotating the pans front to back halfway through, until the chips are golden and just starting to get crispy.

6. Allow the chips to cool in the oven with the heat off and the door propped slightly open. This is a crucial step, as they will be soft initially and crisp up when they cool using this method.

TIPS & VARIATIONS • If you have a dehydrator, you can also make zucchini chips with that. It will take a lot longer, usually at least 8 hours, but sometimes the result is crispier.

• For a flavor twist, try using seasoned salt instead of plain sea salt. You can also add a sprinkle of spices, like paprika, cumin, or dried herbs. Go light on everything, because they will be more concentrated as the chips shrink.

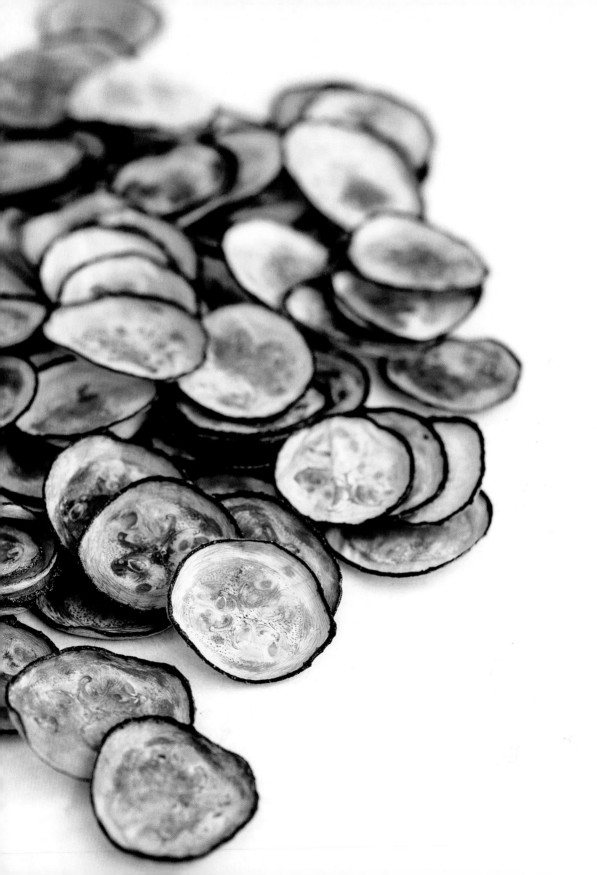

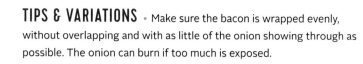

TIPS & VARIATIONS • Make sure the bacon is wrapped evenly, without overlapping and with as little of the onion showing through as possible. The onion can burn if too much is exposed.

• Save the bacon grease for another use, like sautéing veggies.

• When choosing a cooking spray, look for one that is made without chemicals and can withstand high heat, like avocado oil. You can also pour your own oil into a mister.

• If you are dairy-free, you can omit the Parmesan.

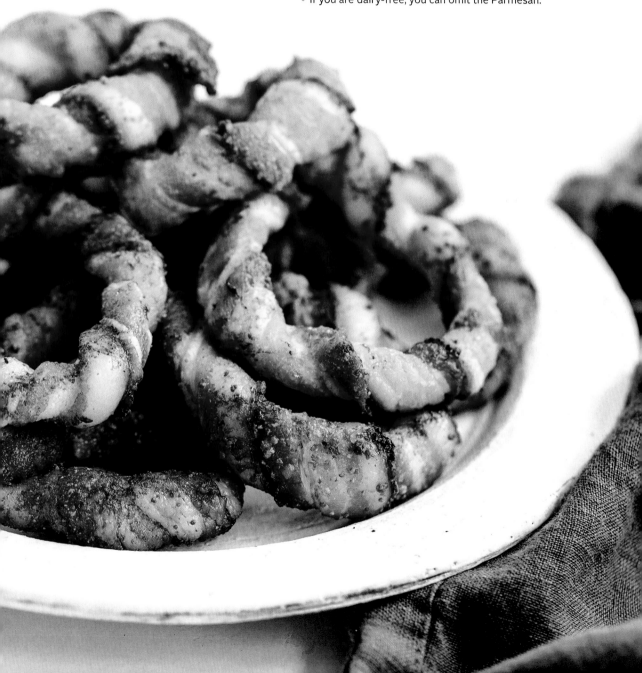

CRISPY BACON WRAPPED ONION RINGS

Traditional onion rings are coated in a thick, high-carb breading. I've experimented with a keto version of the traditional breading (you can find it on WholesomeYum.com!), but wrapping onion rings in bacon is even more delicious. Plus, it's *much* quicker and easier. Can't go wrong with bacon!

1 *extra-large (1 pound)* onion, sliced into ½-inch-thick rings

12 *slices* bacon, halved lengthwise

Avocado oil cooking spray

½ *cup (2 ounces)* grated Parmesan cheese

MAKES 6 SERVINGS

1. Preheat the oven to 400°F. Line a sheet pan with foil. If you have an ovenproof nonstick cooling rack, place it over the pan. (This is optional, but recommended for the crispiest bacon.) Grease the sheet pan or rack.

2. Wrap each onion ring tightly in a thin strip of bacon, trying to cover the whole ring without overlapping. As you finish each ring, place it on a large cutting board in a single layer. (You can also just use the baking sheet without the rack for this step and the next, then use the rack starting at step 5.)

3. Spray the onion rings with avocado oil spray, then sprinkle lightly with half of the grated Parmesan. Flip and repeat on the other side.

4. Place the onion rings on the prepared baking sheet. Bake for 30 to 35 minutes, flipping halfway through, until the bacon is cooked through and starting to get a little crispy on the edges. Drain the bacon grease from the pan occasionally if not using a rack.

5. Switch the oven to broil. Broil the onion rings for 3 to 5 minutes, until crispy. To crisp up more, let the onion rings cool from hot to warm.

SERVING SIZE
⅙ of the onion, 3 to 5 onion rings depending on size (~4 ounces)

PER SERVING
141 calories
8 g fat
7 g total carbs
6 g net carbs
9 g protein

QUICK BITES & SNACKS

MINI SPANAKOPITA BITES

Mini spanakopita bites are inspired by my favorite menu item from a Greek restaurant I worked at in college. Those little triangles of phyllo dough were far from keto-friendly, but they sure were delicious. This recipe makes fathead dough cups stuffed with the same filling you'd find in spanakopita. They are just as satisfying—and perfect for a party!

1. Make the dough through Step 2 of the instructions on pages 17 to 19. If it's too sticky to work with, refrigerate for 30 minutes.

2. Preheat the oven to 350°F. Line 24 cups of a mini muffin tin with parchment paper liners.

3. Use a small (2-teaspoon) cookie scoop to scoop the dough into the cups. Use the back of a teaspoon-size measuring spoon to make a well in the middle of each piece of dough, forming a cup. Dip the measuring spoon in water or oil between each, to prevent sticking. (Alternatively, you can also use your fingers to form the wells.) Make sure the wells are as deep as possible, because the cups will rise and wells will shrink during baking.

4. Bake the empty cups for about 20 minutes, or until firm and golden on the edges.

5. Meanwhile, drain the spinach and squeeze well to get rid of as much water as possible.

6. In a large bowl, stir together the spinach, feta, mozzarella, ricotta, egg, and garlic.

7. When the cups are done baking, scoop the mixture into them. Return to the oven and bake the spanakopita bites for about 10 minutes, until the mozzarella melts.

1 recipe Fathead Dough (page 17)

6 ounces frozen spinach, thawed

⅓ cup (1.7 ounces) crumbled feta cheese

⅓ cup (1.3 ounces) shredded mozzarella cheese

¼ cup (2.2 ounces) full-fat ricotta cheese

1 large egg, whisked

4 cloves garlic, minced

MAKES 24 BITES
(12 SERVINGS)

SERVING SIZE
2 spanakopita bites (2 ounces)

PER SERVING
ALMOND FLOUR VERSION

136 calories
10 g fat
3 g total carbs
2 g net carbs
8 g protein

COCONUT FLOUR VERSION

118 calories
7 g fat
3 g total carbs
2 g net carbs
7 g protein

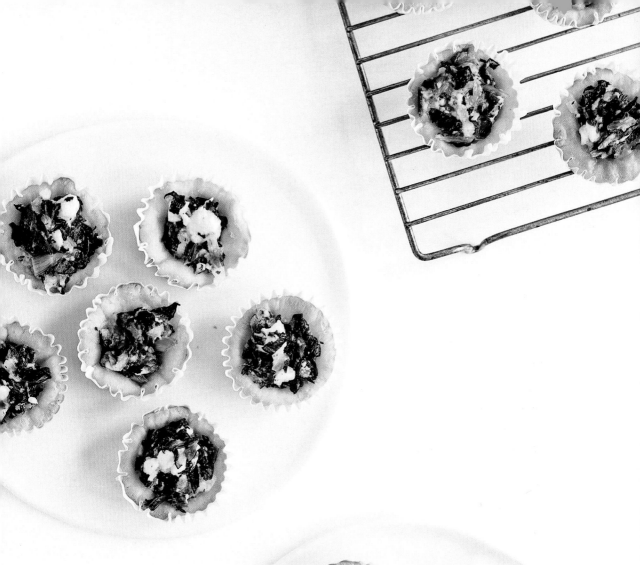

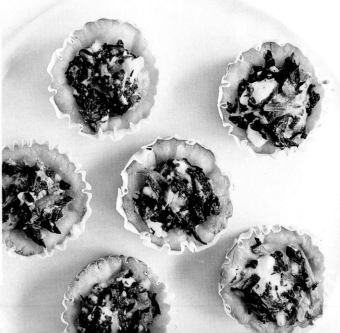

TIPS & VARIATIONS

• If you prefer to use fresh spinach, just cook it first and then squeeze to release water before using it in the recipe.

• Spanakopita bites are a great make-ahead appetizer! You can prepare them and store in the fridge for a few days, or freeze for up to several months. Bake to heat through when you're ready to serve them.

• You can make the same recipe in larger muffin cups, for on-the-go breakfasts or snacks.

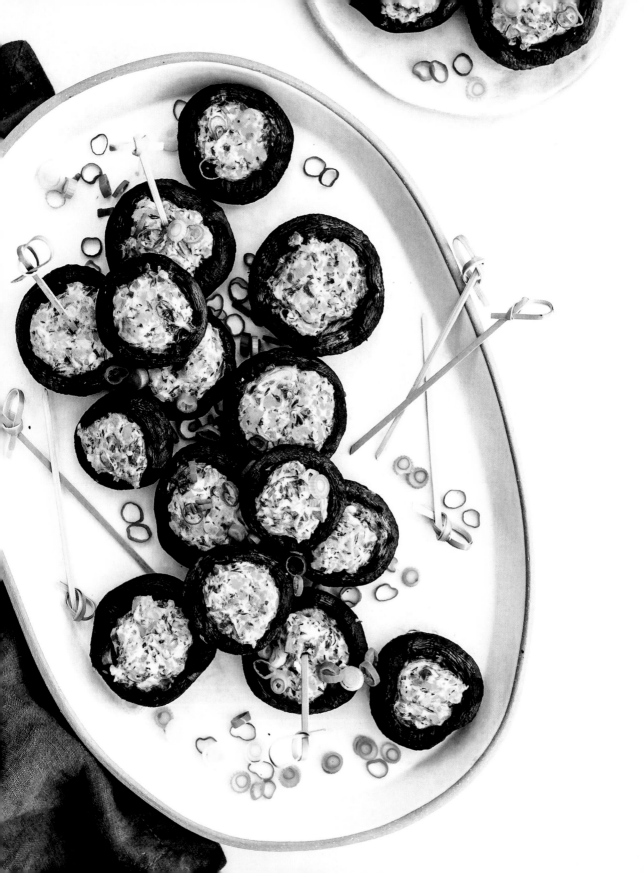

BACON-CHEDDAR DIP STUFFED MUSHROOMS

Stuffed mushroom recipes make a regular appearance at occasions when we're hosting, because they tend to be crowd pleasers and are easy to prepare in advance. These stuffed mushrooms are filled with my favorite dip ever—an indulgent mix of cheeses, ranch seasoning, and bacon. What's not to love?

24 ounces (~7.5 cups) baby portobello mushrooms

2 tablespoons avocado oil

3 ounces (6 tablespoons) cream cheese

¼ cup sour cream

2 cloves garlic, minced

1 tablespoon chopped fresh dill

1 tablespoon chopped fresh parsley

¾ cup (3 ounces) shredded cheddar cheese

⅓ cup cooked bacon bits

3 tablespoons (0.7 ounce) sliced green onions

MAKES 12 SERVINGS

1. Preheat the oven to 400°F. Line a sheet pan with foil or parchment paper and grease lightly.

2. Remove the stems from the mushrooms and place cavity side up on the baking sheet. Drizzle with the avocado oil.

3. Roast the mushrooms for 15 to 20 minutes, until soft.

4. Meanwhile, in a microwave-safe bowl or a saucepan, melt the cream cheese in the microwave or over low heat on the stove until it's soft and easy to stir. Remove from the heat.

5. Stir the sour cream, garlic, dill, and parsley into the cream cheese. Stir in the cheddar, bacon, and green onions.

6. When the mushrooms are soft, remove from the oven but leave the oven on. Drain any liquid from the pan and from inside the mushrooms. Pat the cavities dry with paper towels. Use a small cookie scoop or spoon to fill them with the dip mixture.

7. Bake the stuffed mushrooms for 10 to 15 minutes, until hot.

SERVING SIZE

2 or 3 stuffed mushrooms, depending on size (1.5 ounces)

PER SERVING

107 calories
8 g fat
3 g total carbs
3 g net carbs
4 g protein

TIPS & VARIATIONS • If you don't have fresh herbs on hand, you can use dried. Use 1 teaspoon dried herbs to replace 1 tablespoon fresh.

• Any sharp cheese works well in these mushrooms. Try Swiss, Gruyère, or even pepper jack.

• Stuffed mushrooms can be prepared in advance. Simply leave the last baking step until right before serving.

QUICK BITES & SNACKS

CARAMELIZED ONION MEATBALLS

Both of my kids are obsessed with my mom's *kotleti*—delicious Russian meat patties that use oats as a binder. So naturally, they aren't keto-friendly. These meatballs are inspired by my mom's meat patties, with several changes to make them work with a keto lifestyle. I caramelize the onions she puts in, use almond flour instead of oats, and throw in some fresh herbs for good measure. These are anything but boring meatballs . . . and my kids gobble them up just like my mom's!

1. Preheat the oven to 400°F. Line a sheet pan with foil or parchment paper and grease lightly.

2. In a medium skillet, heat 2 tablespoons of oil over medium heat. Add the sliced onions and cook for at least 20 minutes, until the onions are caramelized and their volume has reduced to about ½ cup. Set aside to cool.

3. Meanwhile, in a large bowl, combine the ground beef, almond flour, egg, rosemary, sage, thyme, sea salt, black pepper, and remaining 2 tablespoons oil. Mix until just combined.

4. When the onions are warm but no longer hot, fold them into the meat until just mixed in. Do not overmix.

5. Using a medium cookie scoop to scoop the meat mixture, gently form balls with your fingertips and place on the lined baking sheet. (You can also use rounded spoonfuls, 1½ to 2 tablespoons in size.)

6. Bake for about 15 minutes, or until almost or just barely cooked through (about 150°F internal temperature). Drain any extra liquid from the pan and wipe the edges of the meatballs if needed.

7. Turn the oven to broil and move the oven rack right under the broiler. Place the meatballs under the broiler for about 2 minutes, until browned.

¼ *cup* olive oil, divided into 2 tablespoons and 2 tablespoons

1¾ *cups (6 ounces)* onion, sliced into thin quarter moons

1 *pound* ground beef

¼ *cup (1 ounce)* blanched almond flour

1 *large* egg

1 *teaspoon* chopped fresh rosemary

1 *teaspoon* chopped fresh sage

1 *teaspoon* fresh thyme, chopped

1 *teaspoon* sea salt

¼ *teaspoon* black pepper

MAKES 18 MEATBALLS (6 APPETIZER SERVINGS)

SERVING SIZE
three 1½-inch meatballs (2.5 to 3 ounces)

PER SERVING
372 calories
29 g fat
3 g total carbs
3 g net carbs
23 g protein

TIPS & VARIATIONS • If you are nut-free, you can replace almond flour with finely ground sunflower seeds.

• It's important not to overmix the meat, because this will lead to tough meatballs.

• Don't try to pack the meatballs tightly when forming them. This will make them dense. Instead, use a cookie scoop and then gently round them with your fingertips.

• The recommended serving size works best as an appetizer, but you can double the serving and serve it over Spaghetti Squash Bolognese (page 108) or Loaded Cauliflower Mash (page 149) for a full meal.

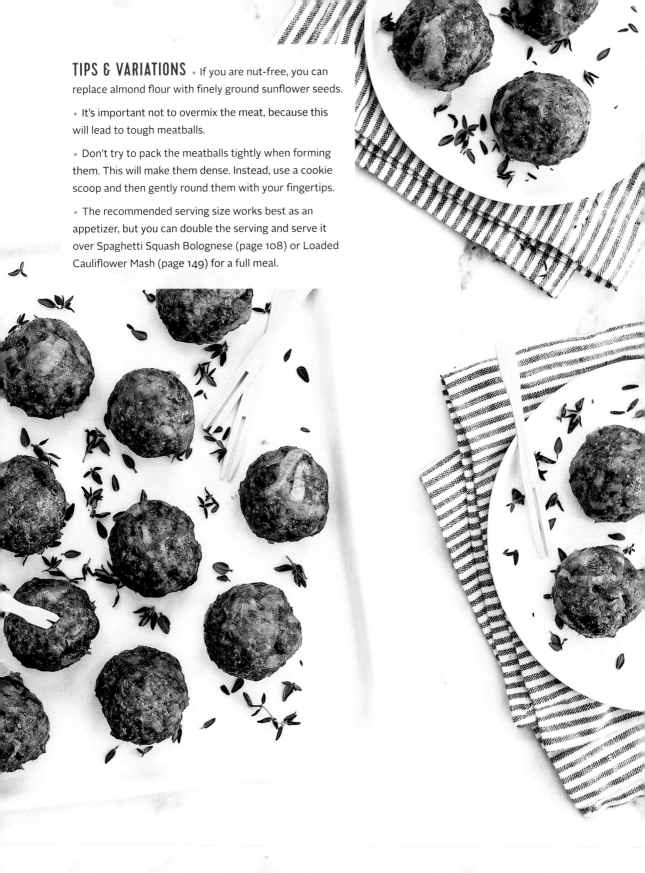

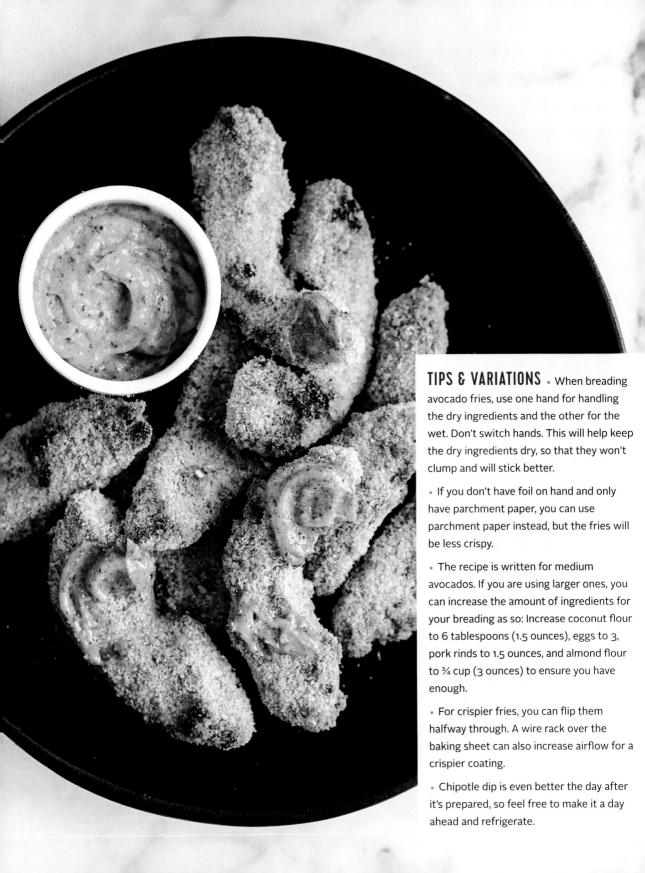

TIPS & VARIATIONS • When breading avocado fries, use one hand for handling the dry ingredients and the other for the wet. Don't switch hands. This will help keep the dry ingredients dry, so that they won't clump and will stick better.

• If you don't have foil on hand and only have parchment paper, you can use parchment paper instead, but the fries will be less crispy.

• The recipe is written for medium avocados. If you are using larger ones, you can increase the amount of ingredients for your breading as so: Increase coconut flour to 6 tablespoons (1.5 ounces), eggs to 3, pork rinds to 1.5 ounces, and almond flour to ¾ cup (3 ounces) to ensure you have enough.

• For crispier fries, you can flip them halfway through. A wire rack over the baking sheet can also increase airflow for a crispier coating.

• Chipotle dip is even better the day after it's prepared, so feel free to make it a day ahead and refrigerate.

CRISPY AVOCADO FRIES WITH CHIPOTLE DIP

Avocado fries make the ultimate keto appetizer, snack, or side dish! They are packed with good fats, loaded with flavor, and very low in carbs. With this recipe, you get a crispy coating on the avocado fries and a zesty chipotle dip to dunk them in.

1. Preheat the oven to 400°F. Line a baking sheet with foil and grease well.

2. **Make the avocado fries:** Halve the avocados lengthwise and remove the pits. Without removing the flesh from the skin, cut parallel lines lengthwise, ¼ to ½ inch apart. Finally, use a large tablespoon to scoop underneath the flesh, separating it from the skin. You'll end up with 4 to 6 slices from each avocado half.

3. In a small bowl, combine the coconut flour, sea salt, and black pepper. In a second small bowl, whisk together the eggs. In a third small bowl, stir together the pork rind crumbs, almond flour, and paprika.

4. Dredge an avocado slice in the coconut flour, dip into the egg, shake off the excess, then press into the "breadcrumb" mixture to coat all sides. Arrange on the baking sheet. Repeat with all the avocado pieces.

5. Bake for about 20 minutes, or until golden. If desired, place under the broiler for 2 to 3 minutes to crisp up more.

6. **Meanwhile, make the chipotle dip:** In a small bowl, whisk together the mayonnaise, lime juice, chipotle powder, and garlic powder until smooth. If you want to adjust the heat, start with less chipotle powder, taste, and then add more, if desired.

AVOCADO FRIES

3 *medium* avocados (6 ounces each)

¼ *cup (1 ounce)* coconut flour

¼ *teaspoon* sea salt

⅛ *teaspoon* black pepper

2 *large* eggs

1 *ounce* pork rinds, crushed to the texture of breadcrumbs

½ *cup (2 ounces)* blanched almond flour

½ *teaspoon* paprika

CHIPOTLE DIP

6 *tablespoons* 2-Minute Avocado Oil Mayonnaise (page 235)

1 *teaspoon* lime juice

½ *teaspoon* chipotle chile powder, or to taste

½ *teaspoon* garlic powder

MAKES 6 SERVINGS

SERVING SIZE

Fries from ½ avocado (4 to 6 fries; 3.25 ounces) + 1 tablespoon dip

PER SERVING

377 calories
33 g fat
14 g total carbs
5 g net carbs
8 g protein

EASY BUFFALO CHICKEN DIP

Buffalo chicken dip is so popular that you'll often find recipes for it on bottles of Buffalo sauce! And it's naturally low carb, as long as you stick to a keto-friendly vehicle for dipping, such as celery. This variation features cheddar and blue cheese, plus heavy cream to make the dip extra creamy.

1. Preheat the oven to 350°F.

2. In a large bowl, stir together the chicken, cream cheese, cheddar, Buffalo sauce, heavy cream, and blue cheese. (It won't fully mix, which is fine.)

3. Transfer the mixture to a shallow 1-quart ramekin or oven-proof appetizer dish. Bake for 20 to 25 minutes, until hot and bubbling.

4. Stir, then either garnish with or stir in the green onions. Serve with low carb veggies, such as celery sticks.

TIPS & VARIATIONS • If you're not a fan of blue cheese, you can replace it with more cheddar instead.

• This makes 16 servings for a crowd, but if you're making it for family, you can cut the recipe in half and use a smaller (16-ounce) ramekin instead. For the recipe as written, a 1½-quart dish will also work, but baking time will be slightly reduced.

• You can make your own shredded chicken in a slow cooker, pressure cooker, or on the stove top, but another option is to buy a rotisserie chicken to save time.

1½ cups (~8 ounces) shredded chicken (rotisserie, or cooked from ~11 ounces raw)

8 ounces (1 cup) cream cheese, cut into 1-inch cubes

1 cup (4 ounces) shredded cheddar cheese

½ cup Buffalo sauce

¼ cup heavy cream

¼ cup (1 ounce) crumbled blue cheese

¼ cup (0.9 ounce) chopped green onions

Celery sticks

MAKES 4 CUPS (16 SERVINGS)

SERVING SIZE
¼ cup (~1.7 ounces)

PER SERVING
120 calories
10 g fat
1 g total carbs
1 g net carbs
6 g protein

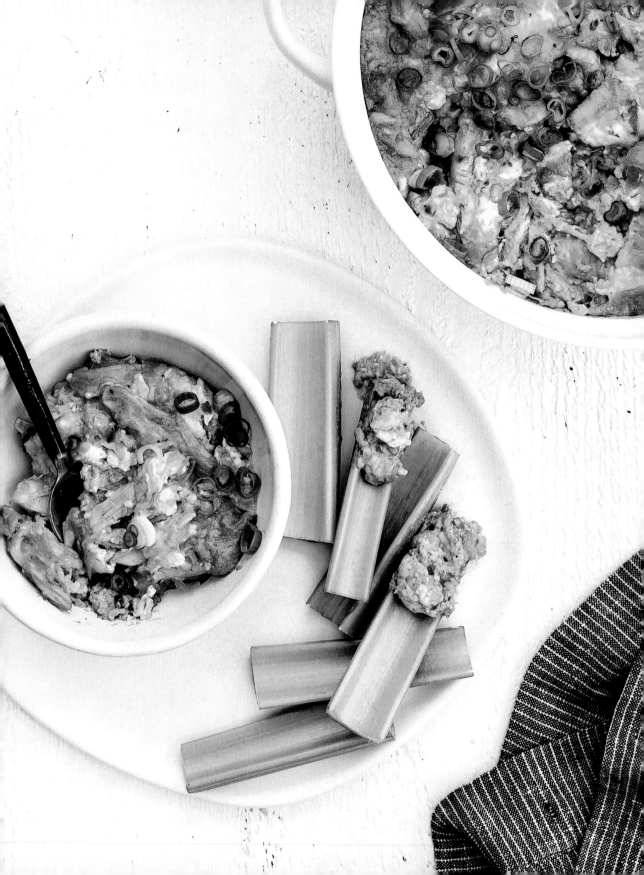

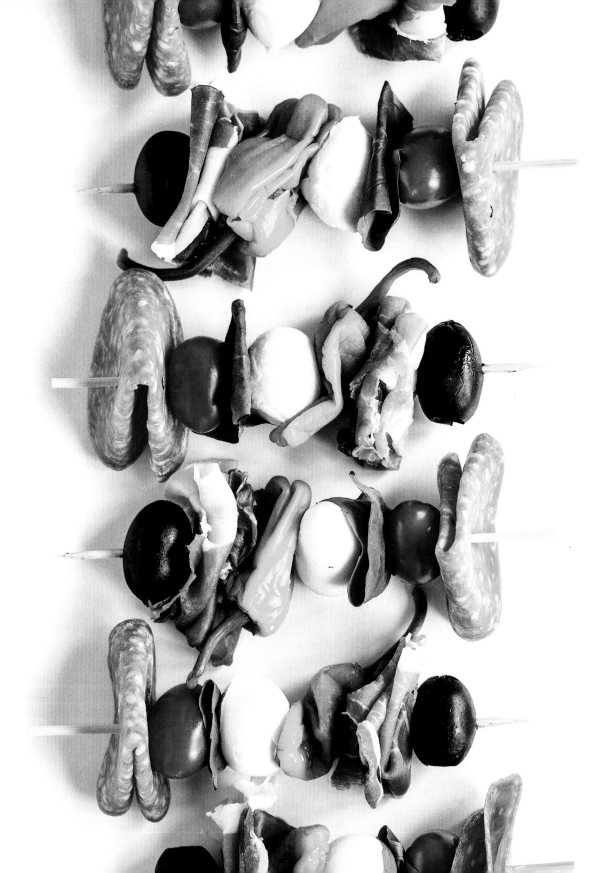

ITALIAN ANTIPASTO SKEWERS

These antipasto skewers were inspired by my husband's love of salami and pepperoncini peppers. He used to get a big antipasto salad packed with both at a pizza place we visited often years ago—a naturally keto-friendly choice way before we started eating that way! I wanted to create an appetizer using those same flavors he loves. Enter Italian antipasto skewers. They are easy to assemble in advance, and they'll please keto and non-keto eaters alike.

Thread the ingredients onto twelve 6-inch skewers in the following order:

- 1 slice salami, folded in quarters (fold in half and fold again)
- 1 grape or cherry tomato
- 1 basil leaf, folded in half with darker side facing out
- 1 mozzarella ball
- 1 pepperoncini pepper (you can prick and drain the liquid first if you'd like)
- 1 half-slice prosciutto, folded a few times to be compact
- 1 olive

12 slices (2.5 to 3 ounces) salami

12 medium (5 ounces) grape or cherry tomatoes

12 medium basil leaves

12 cherry-size (4 ounces) fresh mozzarella balls

12 medium (~4.5 ounces) pepperoncini peppers

6 slices (~3 ounces) prosciutto, cut in half

12 medium (2 ounces) black olives

MAKES 12 SKEWERS (6 SERVINGS)

SERVING SIZE

2 appetizer skewers (3.5 to 4 ounces)

PER SERVING

196 calories
14 g fat
7 g total carbs
4 g net carbs
10 g protein

TIPS & VARIATIONS · The number of skewers you get will vary if yours are not 6 inches long. If they are too short to fit everything, you can make several different kinds in unique combinations.

· Antipasto skewers are super easy to customize! Feel free to leave out any ingredients you don't like, or replace them with something else, like marinated artichokes, green olives, another cheese, or different types of meat.

· Skewers are fun, but you can make this into a salad instead by tossing all the ingredients in a bowl with some oil and vinegar. Cut the basil leaves and meat into smaller pieces for variety.

· For a dairy-free version, simply omit the mozzarella.

VANILLA TOASTED COCONUT CHIPS

Have you ever tried those sweet toasted coconut chips? They can be quite addictive. The problem is, they are too high in sugar for the keto lifestyle. You can easily make your own instead! These toasted vanilla coconut chips make the same convenient sweet snack, without the sugar.

1. Preheat the oven to 325°F. Line a baking sheet with parchment paper.

2. In a medium bowl, whisk together the melted coconut oil, powdered erythritol, vanilla, and sea salt. It may clump, which is okay. Add the coconut chips and toss to coat.

3. Arrange the coconut chips in a single layer on the baking sheet. Bake for about 5 minutes, or until some pieces are starting to turn golden. Stir, then bake for another 3 to 5 minutes, until more golden.

4. Cool completely to crisp up; they will not be crisp right out of the oven.

1 tablespoon coconut oil, melted

2 tablespoons powdered erythritol

½ teaspoon vanilla extract

Pinch of sea salt

2 cups (~6 ounces) unsweetened coconut chips (no other ingredients added)

MAKES 2 CUPS (8 SERVINGS)

SERVING SIZE
¼ cup (~0.75 ounce)

PER SERVING
155 calories
15 g fat
7 g total carbs
2 g net carbs
1 g protein

TIPS & VARIATIONS • For stronger vanilla flavor, scrape half the seeds of a vanilla bean into the coconut oil mixture before tossing with the coconut chips.

• Coconut chips go from golden to burned very quickly, so watch them in the oven carefully. Baking time will vary depending on your oven, rack position, pan, etc.

• Switch it up by trying different spices and extracts, like ½ teaspoon real maple extract and/or cinnamon.

• These coconut chips are just lightly sweet. You can add a little more sweetener if you want them sweeter, but it will be more difficult to mix. Do not add more coconut oil, which will make them too oily.

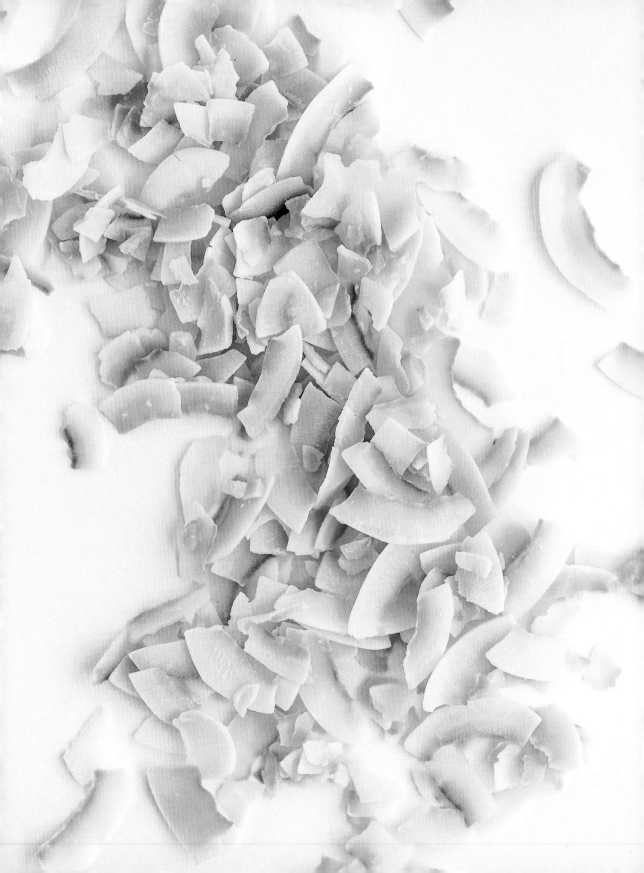

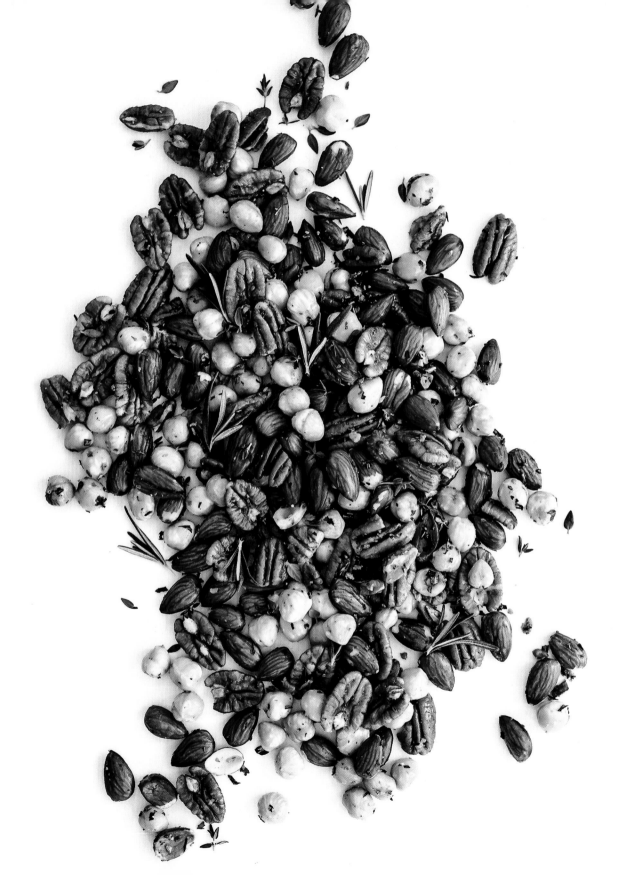

ROASTED GARLIC HERB NUT MIX

Nut mixes are some of the best keto snacks! The key is to portion them out to avoid overeating. Unfortunately, many commercial nut mixes, especially the flavored ones, are filled with hidden carbs and even sugar. No worries—it's super easy to make your own! This roasted garlic herb nut mix is easy to make at home and stores well, so you'll always have some flavored nuts on hand.

1. Preheat the oven to 375°F. Line a baking sheet with foil and grease.

2. In a large saucepan, heat the oil over medium-low heat. Add the rosemary, thyme, oregano, sea salt, garlic powder, and cayenne (if using). Continue to heat for about 2 minutes, until fragrant.

3. Remove from the heat. Add all of the nuts to the pan and stir to coat in the flavored oil and herbs.

4. Spread the nuts on the lined baking sheet in a single layer. Bake for 9 to 12 minutes, stirring about halfway through, until golden.

TIPS & VARIATIONS • For best results, use whole (not pieces of) nuts. Be sure the nuts are raw; already roasted nuts will brown too much in this recipe.

• Almost any kind of raw nuts will work. Almonds, pecans, and macadamias are some of the lowest carb varieties out there, so I chose those. Steer clear of cashews, which have a higher carb count.

- 2 *tablespoons* olive oil
- 1 *tablespoon* finely chopped fresh rosemary
- ½ *tablespoon* fresh thyme, finely chopped
- ½ *teaspoon* dried oregano
- 1 *teaspoon* sea salt
- ½ *teaspoon* garlic powder
- ¼ *teaspoon* cayenne pepper, or to taste (optional)
- 1 *cup* raw almonds
- 1 *cup* raw pecans
- 1 *cup* raw macadamia nuts

MAKES 3 CUPS
(12 SERVINGS)

SERVING SIZE
¼ cup (~1.2 ounces)

PER SERVING
227 calories
22 g fat
5 g total carbs
2 g net carbs
4 g protein

QUICK BITES & SNACKS

BACON GUACAMOLE FAT BOMBS

Fat bombs are often thought of as sweet high-fat treats, but they can be savory, too! The primary ingredients in these fat bombs are two popular staples of the keto lifestyle, avocado and bacon. They are packed with good fats and are excellent for curbing hunger. This also happens to be lower in calories than most fat bomb recipes. It's a win-win!

½ *cup* Simple Guacamole (page 248)

3 *tablespoons* bacon grease, melted

1 *medium* egg yolk, cooked

1 *tablespoon* MCT oil powder (optional)

¼ *cup* cooked bacon bits

MAKES 12 FAT BOMBS

SERVING SIZE
1 fat bomb

PER SERVING
64 calories
6 g fat
1 g total carbs
1 g net carbs
1 g protein

1. In a medium bowl, mash together the guacamole, melted bacon grease, egg yolk, and MCT oil powder (if using).

2. Line 12 cups of a mini muffin tin with parchment paper liners.

3. Scoop about 1 tablespoon of the guacamole mixture into each muffin cup. Place 1 teaspoon bacon bits evenly over the top of each, covering as much of the exposed guacamole as possible, and press gently.

4. Refrigerate for at least 12 hours, until firm.

TIPS & VARIATIONS • You'll need 4 to 6 slices bacon to get the ¼ cup bacon bits and 3 tablespoons bacon grease needed for this recipe. You may need more or less for the bacon grease, depending on the fat content of the bacon you use.

• Like guacamole, these fat bombs may brown a bit on top. Try to cover as much as possible of the top with the bacon bits to help prevent this. They'll keep for 3 to 5 days in the refrigerator.

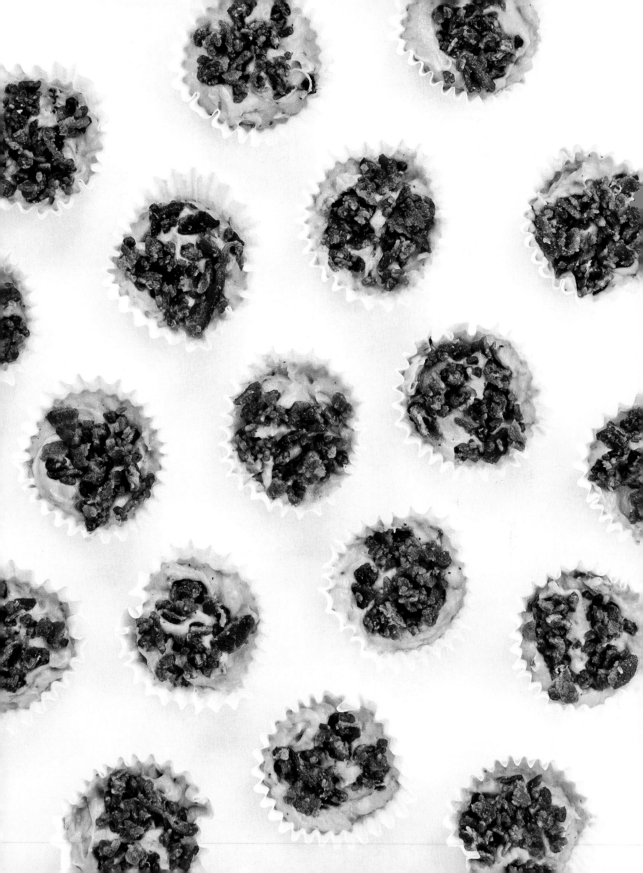

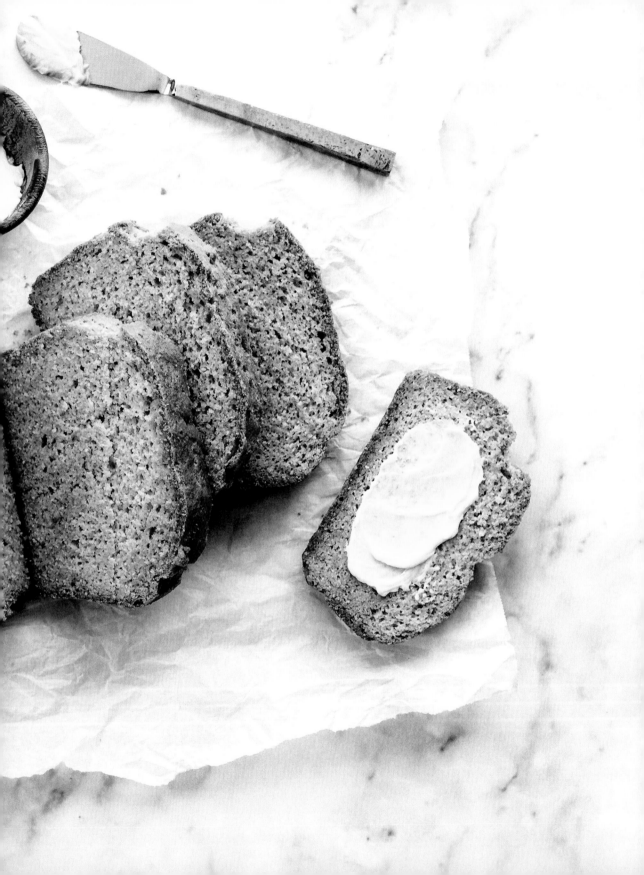

TOO-GOOD-TO-BE-KETO BREADS

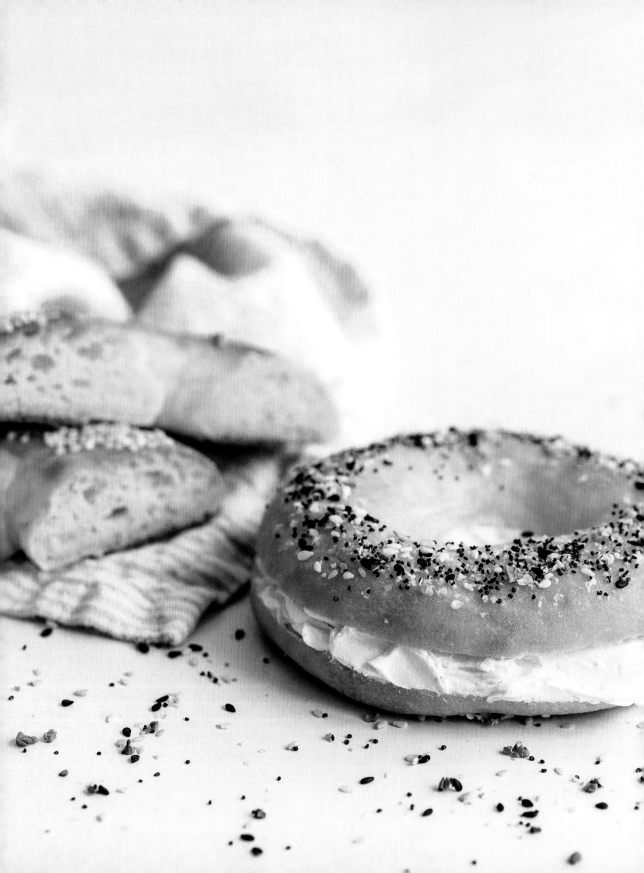

CHEWY FATHEAD BAGELS

I've tested a zillion-and-a-half low carb bread recipes over the years, but I keep coming back to these fathead bagels as my absolute favorite. They are thick and chewy and oh-so-comforting! These are as versatile as traditional bagels—slice and serve with cream cheese, assemble a hearty breakfast sandwich, or even enjoy a bagel sandwich for lunch.

1 *doubled recipe* Fathead Dough (page 17), made with baking powder

1 *tablespoon* sesame seeds, for topping (optional)

MAKES 6 SERVINGS

SERVING SIZE
1 bagel (3.7 ounces)

PER SERVING
ALMOND FLOUR VERSION
386 calories
31 g fat
8 g total carbs
5 g net carbs
20 g protein

COCONUT FLOUR VERSION
313 calories
21 g fat
10 g total carbs
6 g net carbs
19 g protein

1. Make the dough through Step 2 of the instructions on pages 17 to 19. If it's very sticky after being fully incorporated, chill for 30 minutes.

2. Preheat the oven to 400°F. Line a large baking sheet with parchment paper.

3. Divide the dough into 6 portions. On a cutting board, use oiled hands to roll each portion into a long log, then press the ends together to make a bagel shape and place the bagel on the lined baking sheet. The bagels will expand in the oven, so if you want a hole after baking, make it larger than you think you might need. Repeat with the remaining dough, placing the bagels at least 2 inches apart.

4. If using sesame seeds, sprinkle them over the bagels and gently press into the dough.

5. Bake for 10 to 14 minutes, until the bagels are firm and golden.

TIPS & VARIATIONS • If you want extra chewy bagels, add ¼ teaspoon xanthan gum to the dry ingredients when making the dough. They are still pretty chewy without it if you skip it.

• Any bagel toppings you like will work great here. Try "everything" seasoning, which is available at many supermarkets.

• If you haven't worked with fathead dough before, don't miss the tips in the guide (page 16).

TOO-GOOD-TO-BE-KETO BREADS

ALMOND FLOUR BISCUITS

Basic almond flour biscuits are the perfect accompaniment for soups and salads, or simply spread with butter and enjoy with a cup of coffee. You can even make small breakfast sandwiches with them. Plus, they are easy to customize with different flavors.

1. Preheat the oven to 350°F. Line a baking sheet with parchment paper.

2. In a large bowl, mix together the almond flour, baking powder, and sea salt. Stir in the beaten eggs and melted butter to form a dough.

3. Scoop rounded tablespoons of the dough onto the lined baking sheet. (Using a large cookie scoop is the fastest way.) Use the palm of your hand to flatten the biscuits slightly to ¾ to 1 inch thick.

4. Bake for about 15 minutes, or until firm and golden. Cool at least to lukewarm on the baking sheet before enjoying. Biscuits will firm up as they cool.

2 *cups (8 ounces)* blanched almond flour

2 *teaspoons* baking powder

½ *teaspoon* sea salt

2 *large* eggs, beaten

5 *tablespoons +
1 teaspoon (⅔ stick)* butter, melted

MAKES 12 BISCUITS

SERVING SIZE
1 biscuit (1 ounce)

PER SERVING
164 calories
15 g fat
4 g total carbs
2 g net carbs
5 g protein

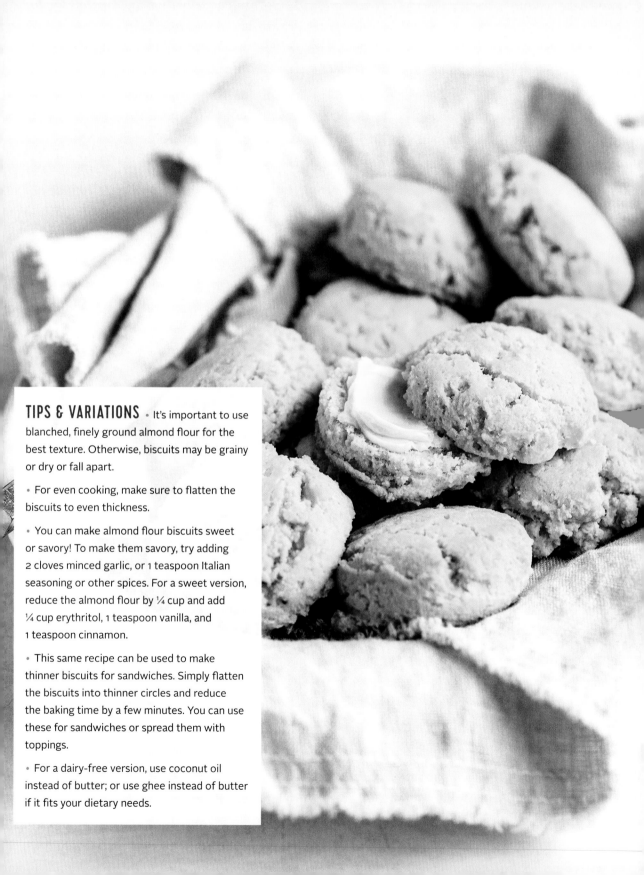

TIPS & VARIATIONS • It's important to use blanched, finely ground almond flour for the best texture. Otherwise, biscuits may be grainy or dry or fall apart.

• For even cooking, make sure to flatten the biscuits to even thickness.

• You can make almond flour biscuits sweet or savory! To make them savory, try adding 2 cloves minced garlic, or 1 teaspoon Italian seasoning or other spices. For a sweet version, reduce the almond flour by ¼ cup and add ¼ cup erythritol, 1 teaspoon vanilla, and 1 teaspoon cinnamon.

• This same recipe can be used to make thinner biscuits for sandwiches. Simply flatten the biscuits into thinner circles and reduce the baking time by a few minutes. You can use these for sandwiches or spread them with toppings.

• For a dairy-free version, use coconut oil instead of butter; or use ghee instead of butter if it fits your dietary needs.

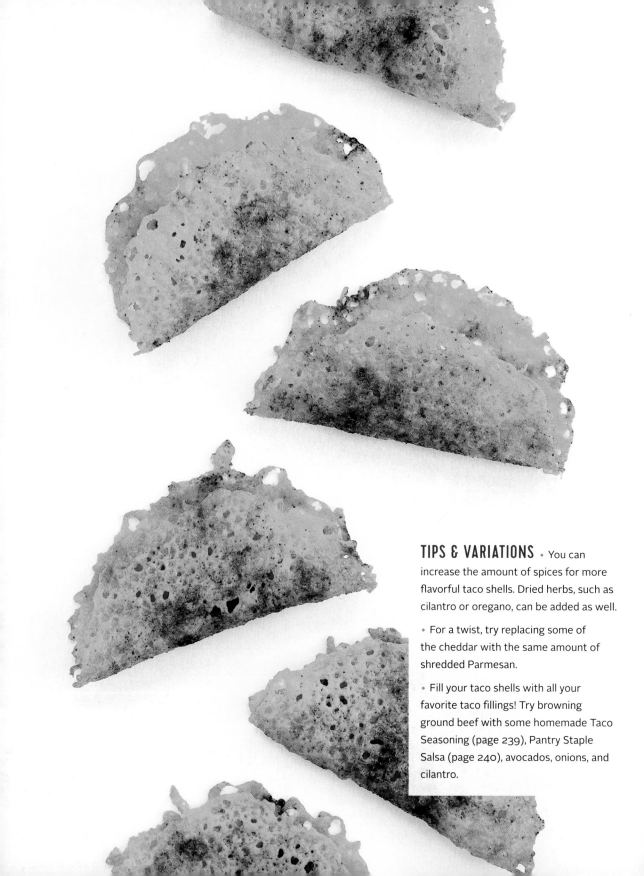

TIPS & VARIATIONS • You can increase the amount of spices for more flavorful taco shells. Dried herbs, such as cilantro or oregano, can be added as well.

• For a twist, try replacing some of the cheddar with the same amount of shredded Parmesan.

• Fill your taco shells with all your favorite taco fillings! Try browning ground beef with some homemade Taco Seasoning (page 239), Pantry Staple Salsa (page 240), avocados, onions, and cilantro.

CHEESE TACO SHELLS

Did you know you can make crispy taco shells out of . . . shredded cheese?! It's so simple. Just bake circles of cheese in the oven along with some spices, then hang them over a spatula so that they harden in the shape of a taco shell. These are a nice change of pace from soft tortillas (though you can make those, too; see page 201).

2⅔ cups (10.7 ounces) shredded cheddar cheese

½ teaspoon ground cumin

¼ teaspoon chili powder

MAKES 8 TACO SHELLS (4 SERVINGS)

SERVING SIZE
2 taco shells (~2.5 ounces)

PER SERVING
152 calories
12 g fat
0 g total carbs
0 g net carbs
9 g protein

1. Preheat the oven to 375°F. Line a baking sheet with parchment paper.

2. Using about ⅓ cup cheddar per taco, sprinkle the cheese on the parchment paper in circles 5 to 6 inches in diameter, with even distribution of cheese throughout each circle. You should be able to fit about 3 circles on the pan. Sprinkle with the cumin and chili powder.

3. Bake for 5 to 7 minutes, until the edges start to brown and the cheese is bubbling vigorously. (It will bubble first, but bake long enough for the edges to brown, too.)

4. Meanwhile, set up 3 wooden spoons or spatulas, with handles at least as long as the diameter of the cheese circles, each sitting horizontally across two upside-down glasses of the same height. This way, they'll be ready once the cheese taco shells are out of the oven.

5. Remove the pan from the oven and let the cheese circles cool on the pan for 1 to 3 minutes, until firm enough to pick up with a spatula without falling apart, but still very soft. Do not let them fully set.

6. Use a flat turner or spatula to lift the cheese circles and hang them over the wooden spoons. Let them hang 5 to 10 minutes, until hardened.

7. Repeat with the remaining cheese to make a total of 8 taco shells.

THE BEST 90-SECOND BREAD

You may have seen 90-second bread recipes floating around. The concept is great, but it's almost too good to be true, and people often complain that it's eggy or crumbly. No more! It's a tall order to call a recipe "the best," but I truly think this is the best 90-second bread—it's sturdy, slightly chewy, and has air pockets, just like real bread. The microwave is the quickest method to make it, but oven instructions are also included if that's your preference.

1. If using the oven method, preheat the oven to 350°F.

2. **Microwave method:** Melt the butter in a 5 × 7-inch glass dish.
   Oven method: In a small saucepan, melt the butter. Pour into an ovenproof 5 × 7-inch glass dish.

3. In a small bowl, stir together the almond flour, psyllium husk powder, baking powder, and sea salt.

4. Add the flour mixture to the melted butter in the baking dish, then whisk in the egg and stir everything together until smooth. Level the top with the back of a spoon.

5. **Microwave method:** Microwave for about 90 seconds, or until firm and springy.
   Oven method: Bake for about 15 minutes, or until firm and springy.

6. Run a knife along the edges, then flip onto a plate or paper towel to release.

7. Cut in half to form 2 thick slices. You can slice each piece in half horizontally for thinner slices, if desired.

8. Toast in a toaster for best results (highly recommended). This improves the texture and reduces any egg-y flavor.

1 *tablespoon* **butter**

3 *tablespoons (0.75 ounce)* **blanched almond flour**

1 *teaspoon* **psyllium husk powder**

½ *teaspoon* **baking powder**

Pinch **of sea salt**

1 *large* **egg**

MAKES 2 SERVINGS

SERVING SIZE

1 slice (1.2 ounces), or ½ the recipe

PER SERVING

150 calories
13 g fat
3 g total carbs
1 g net carbs
5 g protein

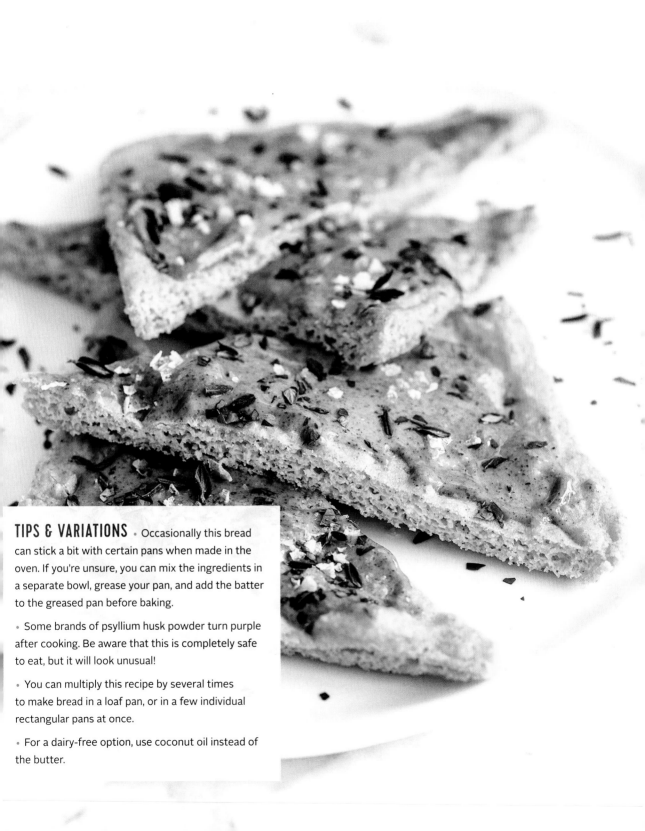

TIPS & VARIATIONS • Occasionally this bread can stick a bit with certain pans when made in the oven. If you're unsure, you can mix the ingredients in a separate bowl, grease your pan, and add the batter to the greased pan before baking.

• Some brands of psyllium husk powder turn purple after cooking. Be aware that this is completely safe to eat, but it will look unusual!

• You can multiply this recipe by several times to make bread in a loaf pan, or in a few individual rectangular pans at once.

• For a dairy-free option, use coconut oil instead of the butter.

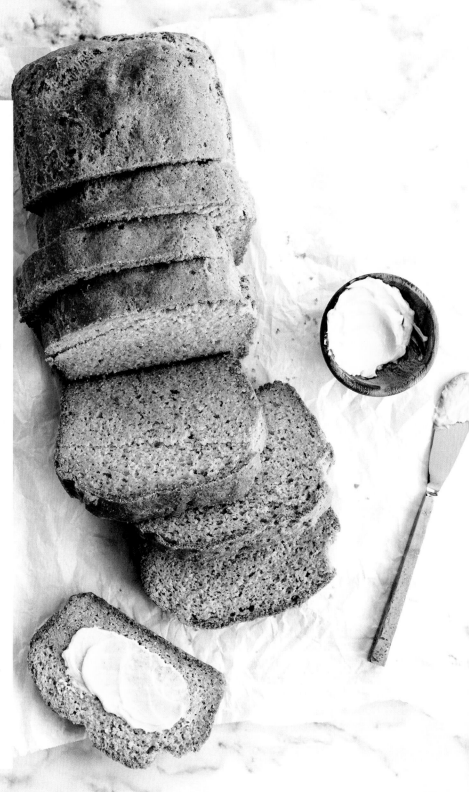

TIPS & VARIATIONS

• The dough can be sticky when transferring it to the pan. To transfer it and round the top, you can use a rubber spatula, but if using your hands, oil them first.

• This bread may pass the toothpick test before it's fully done. To ensure that it's really done, check for other signs of doneness as well. Make sure that the top is also very crusty and the bread doesn't make a squishy sound when pressing on the top.

• Some brands of psyllium husk powder will make the bread turn slightly purple in color after baking. This is just a reaction with the baking powder; it is safe to eat and does not affect the taste, only the appearance. You can try switching brands if it bothers you.

• The serving size for this bread is a pretty thick slice: ½ inch. Depending on your preference, you can easily lighten it up by cutting thinner slices to reduce calories and carbs.

• For a dairy-free option, use coconut oil instead of butter.

EASY ALL-PURPOSE BREAD

Ah, bread: the number one thing people miss with the keto lifestyle. Well, don't miss it—make it! You don't need a complicated recipe or a dozen ingredients. This basic low carb bread will work for just about any use of bread under the sun, and making it is straightforward. It even has a crusty exterior and chewy texture, just like real wheat bread!

3   *cups (12 ounces)* blanched almond flour

⅓   *cup* psyllium husk powder

2   *tablespoons* baking powder

½   *teaspoon* sea salt

6   *large* eggs

½   *cup* unsweetened almond milk

5   *tablespoons +* 1 teaspoon (⅔ stick) butter, melted

MAKES 16 SERVINGS

SERVING SIZE
one ½-inch-thick slice
(~2 ounces)

PER SERVING
203 calories
16 g fat
9 g total carbs
3 g net carbs
7 g protein

1. Preheat the oven to 350°F. Line an 8.5 × 4.5-inch loaf pan with parchment paper, so that it hangs over the two long sides.

2. In a large bowl, stir together the almond flour, psyllium husk powder, baking powder, and sea salt.

3. In another large bowl, with an electric hand mixer, beat the eggs at high speed for 2 to 3 minutes, until doubled in volume. Still at high speed, beat in the almond flour mixture, then the almond milk and melted butter.

4. Press the dough into the lined baking pan. Round the top with your hands or a spatula. (The easiest way is to push the edges down so that they are lower than the center.)

5. Bake for 45 to 55 minutes, until the top is very crusty, an inserted toothpick comes out clean, and you hear no squishy sound when pressing on the top.

6. Cool completely before removing the loaf from the pan.

ITALIAN GARLIC BREAD STICKS

When my husband and I met years ago, he asked me what my favorite restaurant was. My answer? A certain place that serves unlimited salad and bread sticks. I haven't had those bread sticks in years, but thought of them recently and was inspired to create a keto version. They turned out so satisfying! These Italian garlic bread sticks make the perfect addition to soups, salads, or low carb pasta replacements, such as zucchini noodles or spaghetti squash.

1. Make the dough through Step 2 of the instructions on pages 17 to 19, adding the garlic powder to the dry ingredients. Chill the dough for 30 minutes, until it's not too sticky to work with.

2. Preheat the oven to 350°F. Line a baking sheet with parchment paper.

3. Divide the dough into 8 portions. Using oiled hands, shape or roll each into a log about 1 inch thick and 6 to 7 inches long. Place the bread sticks 2 inches apart on the lined pan and flatten slightly.

4. Brush the tops of the logs with the melted butter. Sprinkle with the Italian seasoning and sea salt.

5. Bake the bread sticks for 18 to 22 minutes, until golden.

TIPS & VARIATIONS • Check the fathead dough guide, page 16, for important tips on working with fathead dough.

• Serve bread sticks with low carb pasta, like Spaghetti Squash Bolognese (page 108) or soup, like 5-Ingredient Broccoli-Cheese Soup (page 79).

1 double recipe Fathead Dough (page 17), made with baking powder

1 teaspoon garlic powder

1 tablespoon butter, melted

1 teaspoon Italian seasoning

1 teaspoon sea salt or ½ teaspoon table salt

MAKES 8 SERVINGS

SERVING SIZE
1 bread stick (~2.5 ounces)

PER SERVING
ALMOND FLOUR VERSION
302 calories
24 g fat
6 g total carbs
4 g net carbs
15 g protein

COCONUT FLOUR VERSION
248 calories
17 g fat
7 g total carbs
4 g net carbs
14 g protein

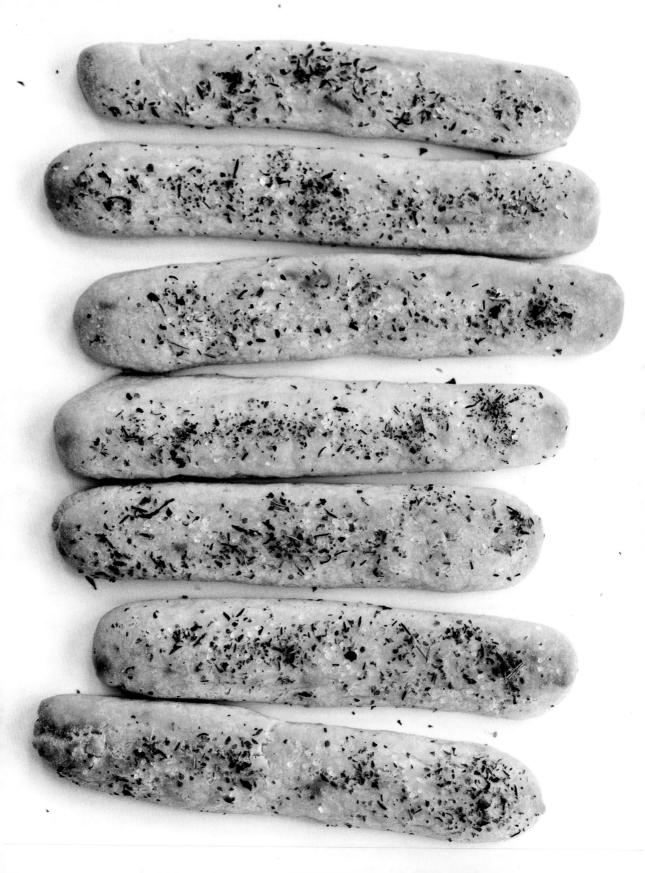

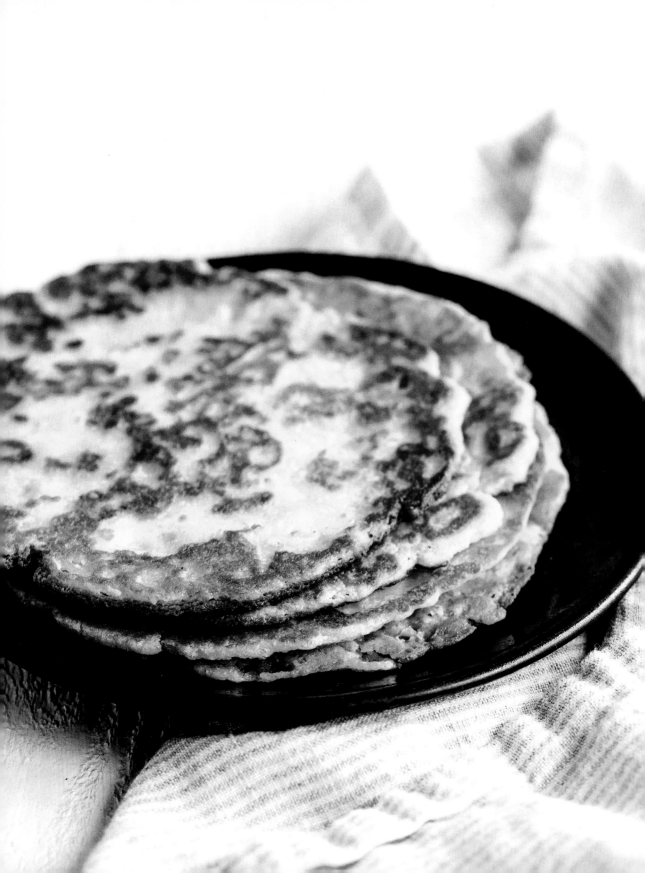

PLIABLE FATHEAD TORTILLAS

Is there anything fathead dough can't do? If you omit the cream cheese, you can make tortillas with it! These keto tortillas take a little practice to get right (check the tips on page 202!), but it's so worth it. Once you have these down, you can make tacos, quesadillas, and more! They also freeze well, so go ahead and make a big batch for later.

1 *double recipe* Fathead Dough (page 17), made without cream cheese

2 *tablespoons* avocado oil (for stovetop method only)

MAKES 4 SERVINGS

SERVING SIZE
two 6-inch tortillas
(~2.25 ounces each)

PER SERVING
ALMOND FLOUR VERSION*
527 calories
42 g fat
10 g total carbs
6 g net carbs
30 g protein

COCONUT FLOUR VERSION*
417 calories
26 g fat
13 g total carbs
6 g net carbs
28 g protein

*Nutrition info does not include oil for cooking if the stovetop method is used.

1. Make the dough through Step 2 of the instructions on pages 17 to 19. If the dough is sticky, chill for about 30 minutes until it's easier to work with. It can be stiff and break apart if you chill it for too long, so if that happens, let it sit at room temperature again to make it more pliable.

2. Divide the dough into 8 portions. Form each piece of dough into a ball and place the ball between 2 greased pieces of parchment paper. Roll each ball into a 6-inch tortilla, ⅛ to ¼ inch thick, or press to this size and thickness using a tortilla press. Repeat with all the pieces of dough.

3. Use a fork to prick holes all over each tortilla, to prevent bubbling during cooking.

STOVETOP METHOD:

4. In an 8-inch skillet, heat a little oil over medium-low to medium heat. Add a tortilla, cover, and cook for about 2 minutes, until the edges start to brown.

5. Flip and cook, covered, for 1 to 2 minutes until golden on the second side.

6. Repeat with the remaining tortillas and oil. Fold or wrap the tortillas while they're warm.

OVEN METHOD:

4. Preheat the oven to 400°F. Line 2 large baking sheets with parchment paper.

recipe continues . . .

5. Place 4 tortillas onto each baking sheet. Use a fork to poke holes in them. Bake for 5 to 10 minutes, until the top starts to get golden. The time will vary significantly based on the exact thickness.

6. Carefully flip and poke a few more holes, especially in any areas bubbling up. Bake for 8 to 10 more minutes, until the top is golden again.

7. Cool to warm before moving the tortillas from the pan. Fold or wrap while warm.

TIPS & VARIATIONS · Check the fathead dough guide, page 16, for important tips on working with fathead dough.

• To make sure the tortillas cook through and to avoid raw dough inside, roll out the tortillas very thin. They won't cook through if they are too thick.

• If you are using the stove top method, make sure the heat is not too high and use a lid, otherwise you'll burn the outside of the tortilla before the inside is done.

• Do not overcook the tortillas. If they get too dark, they will be crispy but will break when you try to fold them.

• Fathead tortillas become less pliable as they cool. If needed, you can reheat them a little in the microwave, or in the oven at low temperature (300°F) to make them softer again.

COFFEE CAKE ZUCCHINI BREAD

Coffee cake zucchini bread is a delectable combination of two common crowd-pleasing sweet treats: coffee cake and zucchini bread! Of course, neither is naturally keto, but this sweet bread is just that. Can you imagine anything better than a moist zucchini bread layered with cinnamon-y coffee cake crumbles?!

1. **Make the zucchini bread:** Place the grated zucchini in a colander over the sink to drain while preparing the other ingredients.

2. Preheat the oven to 350°F. Line a 9 × 5-inch loaf pan with parchment paper, so that the paper is hanging over the two long sides.

3. In a large bowl, with an electric hand mixer, beat together the butter and erythritol on medium speed until fluffy.

4. Beat in the eggs and vanilla. Beat in the almond flour, baking powder, and sea salt, until crumbly.

5. Wrap the grated zucchini in a kitchen towel and squeeze over the sink to release as much water as possible. Stir the zucchini into the bowl. Set aside.

6. **Make the crumble topping:** In a medium bowl, stir together the almond flour, erythritol, cinnamon, and sea salt.

7. In a small bowl, whisk together the melted butter, vanilla, and maple extract (if using).

8. Pour the butter mixture into the almond-cinnamon mixture and either stir to incorporate or use the electric hand mixer at low speed. The mixture should be crumbly.

9. Transfer one-third of the batter from the large bowl into the bottom of the parchment-lined loaf pan. Top with one-third of the crumble topping. Repeat the process two more times,

recipe continues . . .

ZUCCHINI BREAD

1½ cups (8.5 ounces) coarsely grated zucchini

5 tablespoons + 1 teaspoon (⅔ stick) butter, softened at room temperature

¾ cup erythritol

3 large eggs

½ tablespoon vanilla extract

3 cups (12 ounces) blanched almond flour

2 teaspoons baking powder

½ teaspoon sea salt

CINNAMON CRUMBLE

1 cup (4 ounces) blanched almond flour

¼ cup erythritol

1 tablespoon ground cinnamon

Pinch of sea salt

3 tablespoons butter, melted

¼ teaspoon vanilla extract

¼ teaspoon real maple extract (optional, for a brown sugar flavor)

MAKES 12 SERVINGS

creating additional layers of batter and crumble topping, with all the remaining crumble on top.

10. Tent the top of the coffee cake with foil. Bake for 30 minutes.

11. Uncover and continue baking for 35 to 45 minutes, until the top is golden and an inserted toothpick comes out clean.

12. Cool the coffee cake completely in the pan before removing from the pan or cutting.

TIPS & VARIATIONS • About ¼ to ½ cup chopped walnuts or pecans would make a hearty addition to the bread batter.

• For a dairy-free version, use coconut oil instead of butter. However, the texture and flavor is slightly better with butter, with a more tender crumb.

• Wondering why you see so many ingredients in a "10 ingredients or less" book? Many are repeated in this recipe! Even with the layers, I promise it's easy.

SERVING SIZE

one ¾-inch-thick slice (~3.5 ounces)

PER SERVING

313 calories
28 g fat
15 g total carbs
6 g net carbs
10 g protein

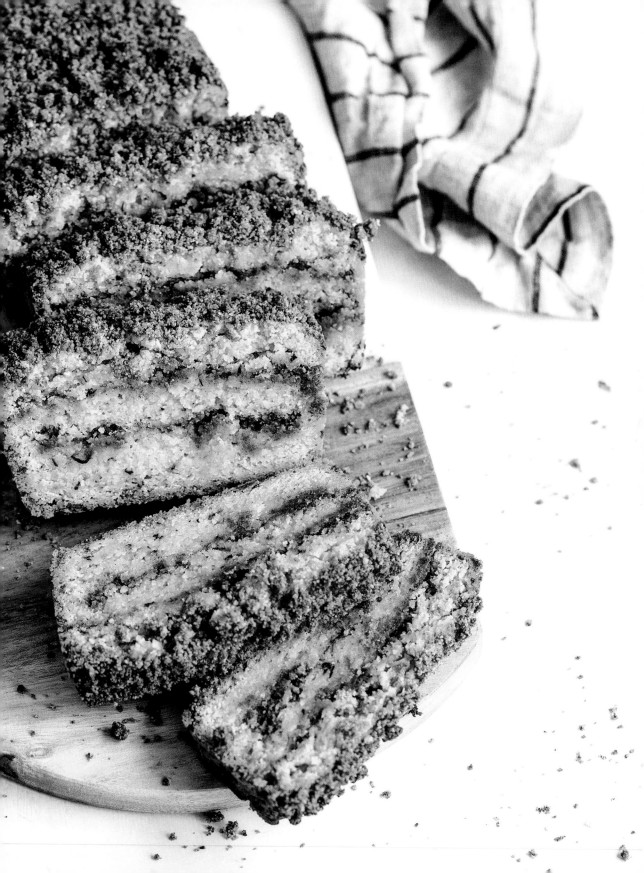

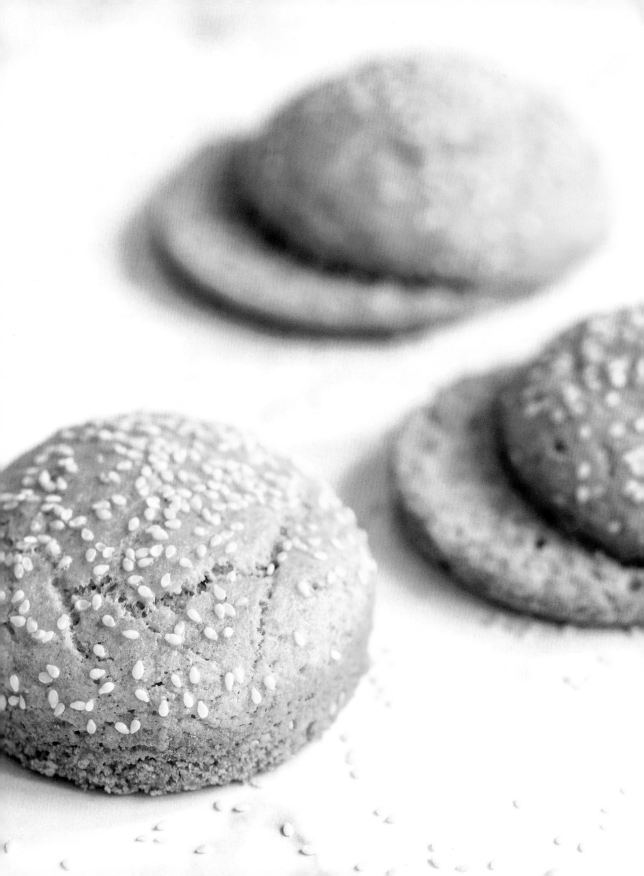

ALMOND FLAX BURGER BUNS

Bunless burgers are great and all, but sometimes it's nice to just hold a burger in your hands! With these almond flour–flaxseed burger buns you can. The addition of gelatin powder makes them chewy, just like regular wheat ones. Pile these buns high with quality meat and your favorite burger fixings.

1 cup (4 ounces) blanched almond flour

⅓ cup golden flaxseed meal

2 tablespoons unflavored gelatin powder

1½ tablespoons baking powder

¼ teaspoon sea salt

3 tablespoons olive oil

3 large eggs, whisked

1 teaspoon sesame seeds

MAKES 4 SERVINGS

SERVING SIZE
1 burger bun (~2.7 ounces)

PER SERVING
403 calories
34 g fat
12 g total carbs
6 g net carbs
16 g protein

1. Preheat the oven to 350°F. Grease the bottom and sides of four 3-inch ramekins.

2. In a large bowl, stir together the almond flour, flaxseed meal, gelatin, baking powder, and sea salt.

3. Stir in the whisked eggs. (You can also whisk eggs directly into the dry mixture if you mix really well.) Add the olive oil and stir again until smooth.

4. Divide the batter evenly among the ramekins. Round the tops slightly by using the back of a spoon to press down along the edges of each ramekin, so that the center is taller. Sprinkle each with ¼ teaspoon sesame seeds and press gently.

5. Bake for 20 to 25 minutes, until golden on top.

6. Let the buns cool completely in the ramekins, then run a knife along the edge and twist to release from the bottom. Slice horizontally in half to use as buns.

TIPS & VARIATIONS · Either regular or golden flaxseed meal will work in this recipe. However, golden has a more neutral flavor that is suitable for burger buns.

· Three-inch ramekins make fairly tall burger buns. If you prefer, you can make wider, shorter buns by using 3½-inch ramekins.

· Instead of sesame seeds, try poppy seeds or "everything" seasoning.

· Use these burger buns for any type of burgers, such as Chili-Lime Turkey Burgers (page 136).

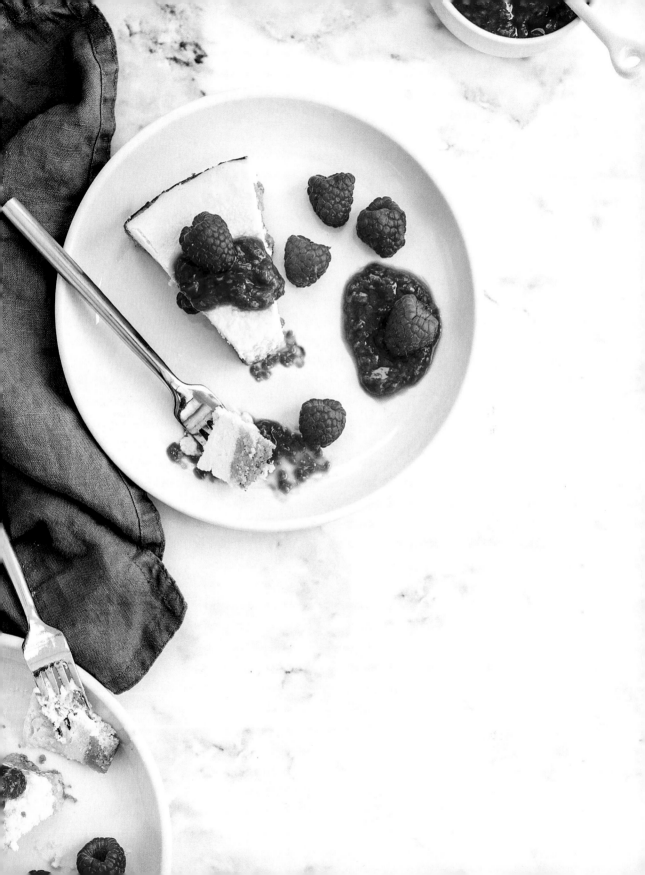

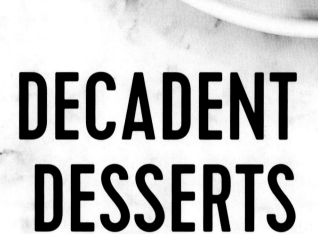

DECADENT DESSERTS

CLASSIC CHEESECAKE

There's a good reason that this cheesecake is the single most popular dessert among Wholesome Yum readers. It tastes exactly like the real thing! It's rich, creamy, and doesn't need a water bath. Enjoy it plain, with Raspberry Sauce (page 244), or with some melted chocolate.

1. Position a rack in the center of the oven and preheat the oven to 350°F. Grease the sides of a 9-inch springform pan and line the bottom with a circle of parchment paper.

2. **Make the almond flour crust:** In a medium bowl, stir the almond flour, melted butter, erythritol, and vanilla until well combined. The dough will be slightly crumbly. Press the dough into the bottom of the prepared pan. Bake for 10 to 12 minutes, until barely golden. Let cool at least 10 minutes. Leave the oven on.

3. **Meanwhile, make the cheesecake filling:** In a bowl, with an electric hand mixer, beat the cream cheese and powdered erythritol together at low to medium speed for about 2 minutes, until fluffy. Keeping the mixer at low to medium the whole time (too high a speed will introduce too many air bubbles, which we don't want), beat in the eggs, one at a time. Finally, beat in the lemon juice and vanilla, scraping down the sides of the bowl periodically.

4. Pour the filling into the pan over the crust. Smooth the top with a spatula (use an icing spatula for a smoother top if you have one). Tap the pan on the counter to release any air bubbles.

5. Bake for 40 to 55 minutes, until the center is almost set, but still jiggly.

6. Remove the cheesecake from the oven. If the edges are stuck to the pan, run a knife around the edge (don't remove the springform edge yet). Cool in the pan on the counter to room temperature, then refrigerate for at least 4 hours, preferably overnight, until completely set. (Do not try to remove the cake from the pan before chilling.)

ALMOND FLOUR CRUST

- 2 *cups (8 ounces)* blanched almond flour
- 5 *tablespoons + 1 teaspoon (⅔ stick)* butter, melted
- 3 *tablespoons* erythritol
- 1 *teaspoon* vanilla extract

CHEESECAKE FILLING

- 32 *ounces (4 cups)* cream cheese, softened at room temperature
- 1¼ *cups* powdered erythritol
- 3 *large* eggs, at room temperature
- 1 *tablespoon* lemon juice
- 1 *teaspoon* vanilla extract

MAKES 16 SERVINGS

SERVING SIZE
1 slice (3.5 ounces), or ¹⁄₁₆ of the recipe

PER SERVING
328 calories
31 g fat
18 g total carbs
5 g net carbs
7 g protein

TIPS & VARIATIONS

• Do not overbake the cheesecake! If you bake it until it's fully set, the result will be dry and crumbly. Instead, you should remove it from the oven when it's still jiggly in the center. It will set after the cooling and chilling process.

• Cheesecake can crack from sudden temperature changes. Make sure to cool completely on the counter before chilling. To be on the safe side, you could bake it in a water bath. Line the outside of the cake pan with foil to keep water out, pour a bit of water into a bigger pan, place the foil-lined pan with the cheesecake inside, then bake. The water reduces temperature changes and therefore cracking, but is an extra step that isn't completely necessary.

• For a nut-free version, try making the crust using coconut flour instead—follow the crust recipe for Key Lime Pie Cupcakes (page 212).

• This recipe commonly has discrepancies when people calculate the carb count, particularly due to the large amount of cream cheese. Cream cheese has 1.56 grams carbs per ounce, but many brands round this up or down, resulting in a discrepancy for the 32 ounces in this recipe.

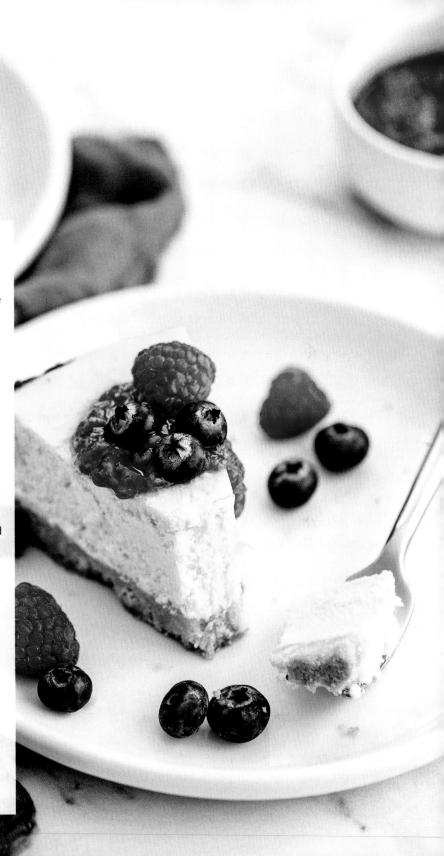

KEY LIME PIE CUPCAKES

Key lime pie offers a great change of pace from the usual chocolate or cake-based desserts. Homemade versions often utilize sweetened condensed milk from a can, but we can achieve a similar result by making our own. I make these mini Key lime pies in a muffin tin to save time and build in some portion control. Don't worry, you still get the same rich, creamy texture and tangy flavor.

1. Preheat the oven to 350°F. Line 12 cups of a muffin tin with paper liners.

2. **Make the crust:** In a large bowl, stir together the coconut flour and erythritol. Stir in the melted butter and egg, until evenly combined. The dough will be crumbly, but you should be able to pinch it together.

3. Press a thin layer of the dough into the bottoms of the lined muffin cups. Bake for 10 to 12 minutes, until firm and slightly golden on the edges. Set aside to cool.

4. **Meanwhile, make the filling:** In a large sauté pan (not a saucepan), melt the butter over medium heat. Whisk in the heavy cream and powdered erythritol to combine. Bring to a boil, then reduce to a simmer and simmer for 30 to 45 minutes, stirring occasionally, until the mixture is thick, coats the back of a spoon, and the volume is reduced by half. It will also pull away from the pan as you tilt it. (This process will go faster if you use a larger pan.) Remove from the heat and set aside to cool for about 10 minutes, until warm but no longer hot. Meanwhile, preheat the oven to 350°F again.

5. Stir the sour cream, lime zest, lime juice, and vanilla into the condensed milk.

6. Pour the filling into the muffin cups over the crust, which should have cooled enough and no longer be hot.

7. Return the pan to the oven for 5 to 10 minutes, until bubbles

CRUST

¾ *cup (3 ounces)* coconut flour

2 *tablespoons* erythritol

4 *tablespoons (½ stick)* butter, melted

2 *large* eggs

FILLING

6 *tablespoons (¾ stick)* butter

3 *cups* heavy cream

¾ *cup* powdered erythritol

½ *cup* sour cream

1 *tablespoon* lime zest, plus more for garnish (optional)

½ *cup* lime juice

1 *teaspoon* vanilla extract

Sugar-free whipped cream, for garnish (optional)

MAKES 12 CUPCAKES

SERVING SIZE
1 cupcake
(~2.7 ounces)

PER SERVING
337 calories
33 g fat
16 g total carbs
4 g net carbs
3 g protein

form on top and the cupcakes start to set on the edges but not in the center. Do not let the filling fully set or brown.

8. Remove the pan from the oven and cool completely on the counter, then chill for at least 1 to 2 hours, until set. (If possible, chilling overnight is even better.)

9. If desired, top with sugar-free whipped cream and/or additional lime zest.

TIPS & VARIATIONS • I used regular limes for this recipe because they are easier to find, but if you can find Key limes, even better. Alternatively, lime juice from a bottle works fine as well, but the zest should be fresh.

• If you squeeze fresh lime juice, you'll have extra zest left over. This makes a great garnish for the cupcakes. Or you can also save it for other uses, such as whisking into salad dressing.

• Try to use the largest sauté pan you can find for making the sweetened condensed milk in step 4. The larger the pan, the faster the condensed milk will form. Don't use a saucepan, which can take hours with this volume of ingredients.

• Be careful not to overbake the filling, otherwise the finished result will not have the smooth texture of Key lime pie. The sign of doneness is tiny bubbles forming on top, but the filling should not be firm or set.

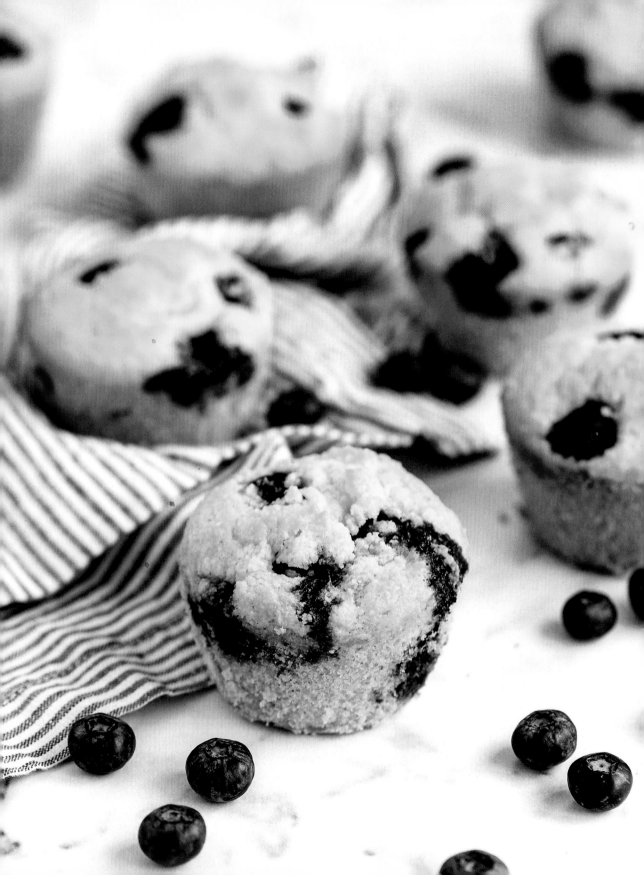

BLUEBERRY MUFFINS

I've never been much of a morning person, but interestingly enough, a productive morning with a steaming cup of coffee is one of my favorite things in the world. The only thing better? Adding a warm blueberry muffin to the mix. These are rich and moist with a delicate crumb, just like traditional blueberry muffins.

2½ cups (10 ounces) blanched almond flour

½ cup erythritol

1½ teaspoons baking powder

¼ teaspoon sea salt

⅓ cup coconut oil, melted

⅓ cup unsweetened almond milk

3 large eggs

½ teaspoon vanilla extract

¾ cup (2.6 ounces) blueberries

MAKES 10 MUFFINS

1. Preheat the oven to 350°F. Line 10 cups of a muffin tin with silicone or parchment paper liners.

2. In a large bowl, stir together the almond flour, erythritol, baking powder, and sea salt.

3. Stir in the melted coconut oil, almond milk, eggs, and vanilla. Fold in the blueberries.

4. Distribute the batter evenly among the muffin cups. Bake for about 25 minutes, until the tops are golden and an inserted toothpick comes out clean.

SERVING SIZE
1 muffin (~2.5 ounces)

PER SERVING
254 calories
23 g fat
11 g total carbs
5 g net carbs
8 g protein

TIPS & VARIATIONS • This recipe is naturally dairy-free. However, if you don't mind dairy, replacing the coconut oil with butter adds a really nice flavor.

• You can use frozen blueberries if you'd like, but do not thaw them. Place them in the batter frozen. If you thaw them, the muffins will be too wet.

• If you want nice muffin tops, this recipe makes 10 muffins. However, if you want to stretch the macros per muffin, you can also prepare it for 12, instead—you'll just have flatter muffins. The nutrition info is assuming 10 muffins, but will be less if you make 12.

• These also work well as mini muffins. You'll get 20 to 24 mini muffins, depending on how high you fill the cups with batter. The baking time will be reduced to about 20 minutes.

FUDGY BROWNIES

Brownie lovers typically fall into two camps: those who like a fudgy brownie, and those who like them lighter and cakier. I'm definitely in the first camp—I'm a firm believer that brownies should be dense and super-chocolaty, and this recipe yields just that.

1. Preheat the oven to 350°F. Line an 8-inch square pan with parchment paper, with the edges of the paper over two of the sides.

2. In a double boiler top or heatproof bowl, combine the butter and chocolate. Bring water to a simmer in the bottom part of the double boiler or a saucepan. Place the double boiler top or bowl over the simmering water and heat gently, stirring frequently.

3. Remove the bowl from the pan as soon as the chocolate pieces have all melted and stir in the vanilla, if desired.

4. Add the almond flour, powdered erythritol, cocoa powder, sea salt, and eggs. Stir together until uniform. The batter will be a little grainy looking.

5. Transfer the batter to the lined pan. Smooth the top with a spatula or the back of a spoon. If desired, sprinkle with the chopped walnuts and press into the top.

6. Bake for 15 to 20 minutes, until an inserted toothpick comes out almost clean with just a little batter on it that balls up between your fingers. (Do *not* wait for it to come out totally clean. Do *not* wait for the brownies to be totally firm or completely set. Do *not* pour off any liquid pooled on top.)

7. Cool completely before moving or cutting. (Do *not* cut while warm.) Use the overhanging pieces of parchment paper to lift the uncut brownies out of the pan and place on a cutting board. Cut into 16 brownies using a straight-down motion, not a seesaw motion, and wipe the knife between cuts if you notice sticking. These brownies are even better the next day!

½ cup (1 stick) butter

4 ounces unsweetened baker's chocolate

1 teaspoon vanilla extract (optional)

¾ cup (3 ounces) blanched almond flour

⅔ cup powdered erythritol

2 tablespoons unsweetened cocoa powder

¼ teaspoon sea salt (only if using unsalted butter)

2 large eggs, at room temperature, whisked

¼ cup walnuts, chopped (optional)

MAKES 16 BROWNIES

SERVING SIZE
1 brownie (~1.5 ounces), or ¹⁄₁₆ of the pan

PER SERVING*
163 calories
15 g fat
6 g total carbs
1 g net carbs
2 g protein

*Nutrition info does not include optional walnuts.

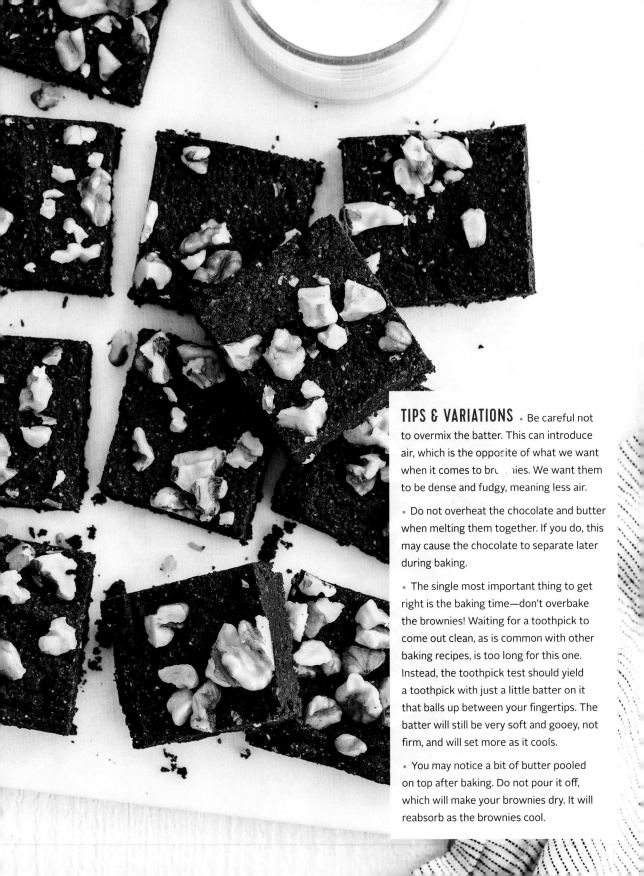

TIPS & VARIATIONS

• Be careful not to overmix the batter. This can introduce air, which is the opposite of what we want when it comes to brownies. We want them to be dense and fudgy, meaning less air.

• Do not overheat the chocolate and butter when melting them together. If you do, this may cause the chocolate to separate later during baking.

• The single most important thing to get right is the baking time—don't overbake the brownies! Waiting for a toothpick to come out clean, as is common with other baking recipes, is too long for this one. Instead, the toothpick test should yield a toothpick with just a little batter on it that balls up between your fingertips. The batter will still be very soft and gooey, not firm, and will set more as it cools.

• You may notice a bit of butter pooled on top after baking. Do not pour it off, which will make your brownies dry. It will reabsorb as the brownies cool.

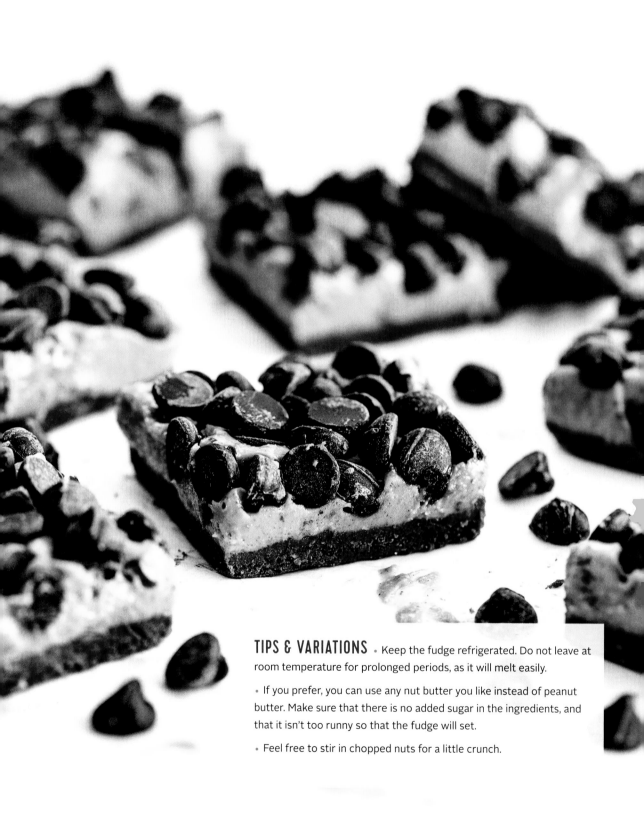

TIPS & VARIATIONS • Keep the fudge refrigerated. Do not leave at room temperature for prolonged periods, as it will melt easily.

• If you prefer, you can use any nut butter you like instead of peanut butter. Make sure that there is no added sugar in the ingredients, and that it isn't too runny so that the fudge will set.

• Feel free to stir in chopped nuts for a little crunch.

CHOCOLATE PEANUT BUTTER CUP FUDGE

You know the phrase "go together like peanut butter and jelly"? Well, I prefer things that go together like peanut butter and chocolate! That combination is way better. This easy recipe is like a cross between fudge and a peanut butter cup, without the fuss of making individual cups.

1. Line an 8-inch square baking dish with parchment paper, letting it hang over two of the sides. Set aside.

2. **Make the chocolate layer:** In a bowl, with an electric hand mixer, beat the butter and powdered erythritol together at medium speed, just until fluffy and combined.

3. Beat in the cocoa powder, vanilla, and sea salt. Adjust sweetener to taste. Do not overmix.

4. Transfer the mixture to the lined baking dish. Smooth the top with a spatula or spoon. Place in the refrigerator while you make the next layer.

5. **Make the peanut butter layer:** In a separate bowl, with an electric hand mixer, beat together the peanut butter, butter, powdered erythritol, peanut butter powder, and vanilla at medium speed. Adjust sweetener to taste.

6. Take the pan out of the refrigerator. Spread the peanut butter mixture over the chocolate. Top with the chocolate chips and press gently.

7. Refrigerate for at least 2 hours, or overnight, until firm.

8. Run a knife along the edge and pull out using the edges of the parchment paper. Slice carefully into sixteen 2-inch squares for a filling dessert, or sixty-four 1-inch squares for mini fat bombs.

CHOCOLATE LAYER

- 1½ cups (3 sticks) butter, softened at room temperature
- 6 tablespoons powdered erythritol
- 6 tablespoons unsweetened cocoa powder
- 1½ teaspoons vanilla extract
- ⅛ teaspoon sea salt

PEANUT BUTTER LAYER

- 1½ cups creamy salted peanut butter (not too runny, no sugar added)
- 6 tablespoons (¾ stick) butter, softened at room temperature
- 6 tablespoons powdered erythritol
- ⅓ cup peanut butter powder
- 1½ teaspoons vanilla extract
- 1½ cups sugar-free chocolate chips

MAKES 16 DESSERT SERVINGS OR 64 FAT BOMB SERVINGS

SERVING SIZE
one 2-inch dessert square (~2.5 ounces) or one 1-inch fat bomb square (~0.6 ounces)

PER DESSERT SERVING	PER FAT BOMB SERVING
400 calories	100 calories
39 g fat	10 g fat
19 g total carbs	5 g total carbs
7 g net carbs	2 g net carbs
9 g protein	2 g protein

SALTED PECAN FAT BOMBS

Salted pecan fat bombs taste like a sweet, decadent dessert, but they have no sugar and can help you hit your desired fat macro ratio on a keto lifestyle. They are also very satisfying! I keep a big batch of these in the fridge to squash cravings when they strike.

1. Line 24 cups of a mini muffin tin with paper liners.

2. In a large sauté pan (not a saucepan!), heat the butter and the sweetener over medium heat for 5 to 8 minutes, stirring frequently, until dark golden brown.

3. Add the cream and sea salt. Bring to a gentle simmer, then simmer for 15 to 20 minutes, until dark golden and thick.

4. Remove from the heat and allow the caramel to cool for a few minutes. Stir in the vanilla and chopped pecans.

5. Scoop the mixture into the lined mini muffin cups, about 1 tablespoon in each. If desired, sprinkle with sea salt. Gently press 1 whole pecan into the top of each.

6. Let the fat bombs cool to room temperature first, then refrigerate for at least 1 hour, or overnight, until set.

TIPS & VARIATIONS • Store pecan fat bombs in the fridge for about 1 week, or freeze for several months.

• For a pecan pie flavor, add ¼ teaspoon real maple extract to the caramel sauce at the end.

• You can make this recipe with any kind of nuts you like. Macadamia nuts or almonds are also great options for the keto lifestyle.

1 *cup (2 sticks)* butter

¾ *cup* powdered monk fruit sweetener blend (1:1 powdered sugar replacement)

1 *cup* heavy cream

1 *teaspoon* sea salt, plus more for sprinkling (optional)

1 *teaspoon* vanilla extract

2 *cups* coarsely chopped pecans

24 whole pecans

MAKES 24 SERVINGS

SERVING SIZE
1 fat bomb (1 ounce)

PER SERVING
171 calories
18 g fat
7 g total carbs
1 g net carbs
1 g protein

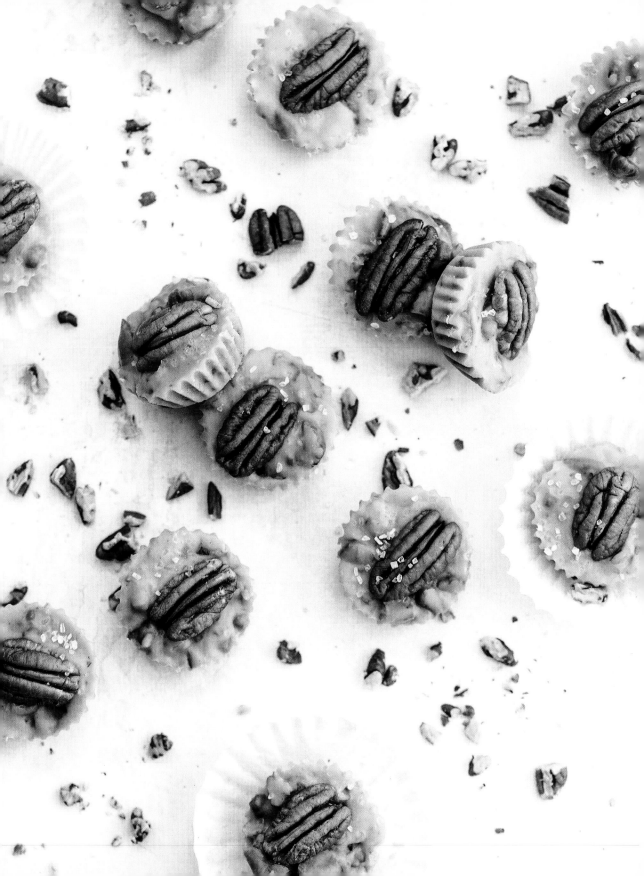

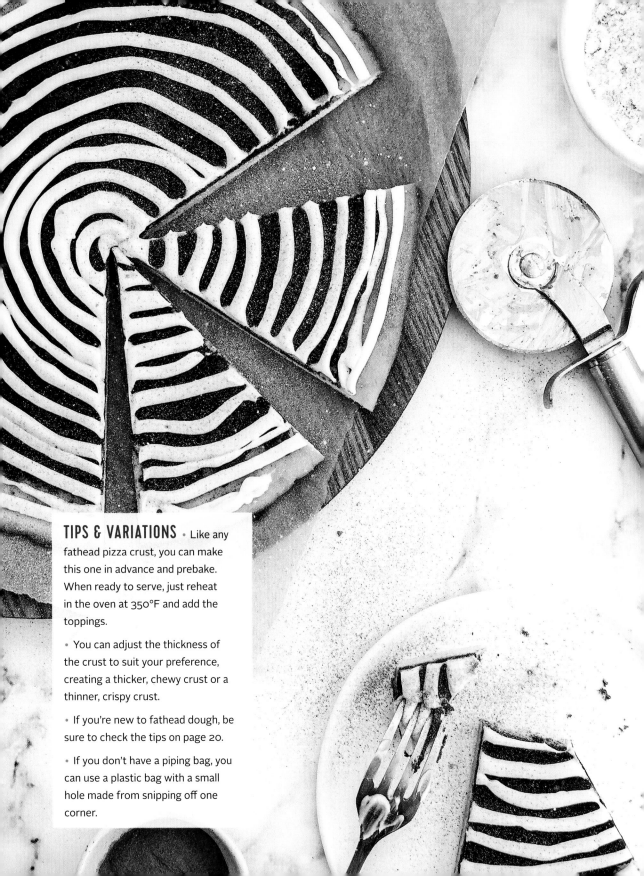

TIPS & VARIATIONS • Like any fathead pizza crust, you can make this one in advance and prebake. When ready to serve, just reheat in the oven at 350°F and add the toppings.

• You can adjust the thickness of the crust to suit your preference, creating a thicker, chewy crust or a thinner, crispy crust.

• If you're new to fathead dough, be sure to check the tips on page 20.

• If you don't have a piping bag, you can use a plastic bag with a small hole made from snipping off one corner.

CINNAMON ROLL DESSERT PIZZA

If you like Fathead Pizza Crust (page 99), you're going to love this sweet version! It's like a giant cinnamon roll, on the same chewy crust, but lightly sweetened. The cinnamon roll topping and icing has all the flavors of your favorite sweet rolls.

1. Make the dough through Step 2 of the instructions on pages 17 to 19. Refrigerate the dough for 30 minutes, until no longer sticky.

2. Preheat the oven to 400°F.

3. When the dough has chilled enough to handle, place it between 2 oiled pieces of parchment paper and roll it out to a circle, about ¼ inch thick and 10 inches in diameter.

4. Slide the parchment paper with the crust onto a pizza stone or pizza pan. Poke holes all over with a fork. Bake for 8 to 10 minutes, until golden.

5. **Meanwhile, make the cinnamon butter:** To prevent seizing, let the melted butter cool for a couple of minutes before adding the other ingredients. In a small bowl, whisk together the melted butter, powdered erythritol, and cinnamon.

6. When the crust is golden, remove it from the oven, and let cool for a few minutes. Then spread the cinnamon butter over it.

7. **Make the icing:** In a deep bowl, with an electric hand mixer, beat the softened cream cheese and butter until fluffy. Beat in the powdered erythritol and vanilla until smooth. Add the heavy cream and beat again. If it's too thick, add more cream until the desired consistency for icing is reached. Adjust the sweetener to taste if needed.

8. Let the pizza cool for at least 10 minutes before adding the icing. Place the icing in a piping bag and pipe in a swirl pattern like a big cinnamon roll.

CRUST

1 recipe Fathead Dough (page 17), made with sweetener

CINNAMON BUTTER

4 tablespoons (½ stick) butter, melted

¼ cup powdered erythritol

1 tablespoon cinnamon

ICING

1.5 ounces (3 tablespoons) cream cheese, softened

½ tablespoon butter, softened

3 tablespoons powdered erythritol

½ teaspoon vanilla extract

2 tablespoons heavy cream, plus more as needed

MAKES 8 SERVINGS

SERVING SIZE

1 slice (2.25 ounces), or ⅛ of entire pizza

PER SERVING
ALMOND FLOUR VERSION

236 calories
21 g fat
13 g total carbs
3 g net carbs
8 g protein

COCONUT FLOUR VERSION

209 calories
17 g fat
13 g total carbs
3 g net carbs
7 g protein

HAZELNUT ICE CREAM

I stick to eating mostly keto when at home, but I like to treat myself to international cuisine when I travel. This keto-friendly hazelnut ice cream is inspired by travels to France and Italy, where hazelnut ice cream and gelato is available everywhere you turn.

1⅓ cups blanched hazelnuts, divided into 1 cup whole and ⅓ cup coarsely chopped

1½ cups unsweetened vanilla almond milk

½ cup powdered erythritol

4 large egg yolks

1½ cups heavy cream

MAKES 2½ CUPS (5 SERVINGS)

SERVING SIZE
½ cup (4 ounces)

PER SERVING
349 calories
35 g fat
18 g total carbs
3 g net carbs
5 g protein

1. In a food processor or high-powered blender, pulse 1 cup of the whole hazelnuts, scraping down the sides frequently, until it reaches a nut flour consistency.

2. Transfer the hazelnut flour to a large saucepan. Stir in the almond milk and powdered erythritol, and bring to a boil over medium heat. Remove from the heat.

3. In a medium bowl, whisk the egg yolks until smooth. Slowly pour the mixture from the saucepan into the yolks while whisking constantly. This is called tempering and needs to be done slowly to avoid cooking the eggs in the process.

4. Return the mixture to the saucepan and cook over low heat for about 10 minutes, stirring frequently, until the mixture coats the back of a spoon. Keep the heat very low and watch closely to avoid curdling.

5. Pour the mixture into a cheesecloth-lined strainer set over a large bowl and squeeze all the liquid into the bowl (about 1 cup). Cool for about 10 minutes, until warm but no longer hot.

6. Stir the heavy cream into the bowl.

7. Transfer the mixture to an ice cream maker and process according to the manufacturer's instructions. (For most ice cream makers, you'll turn the ice cream maker on, pour the mixture into the frozen freezer bowl, and let it mix until thickened, 15 to 20 minutes.)

8. Five minutes before the churning is completed, add the ⅓ cup chopped hazelnuts and let them mix in completely. Transfer to a container and freeze for at least 4 hours, until firm.

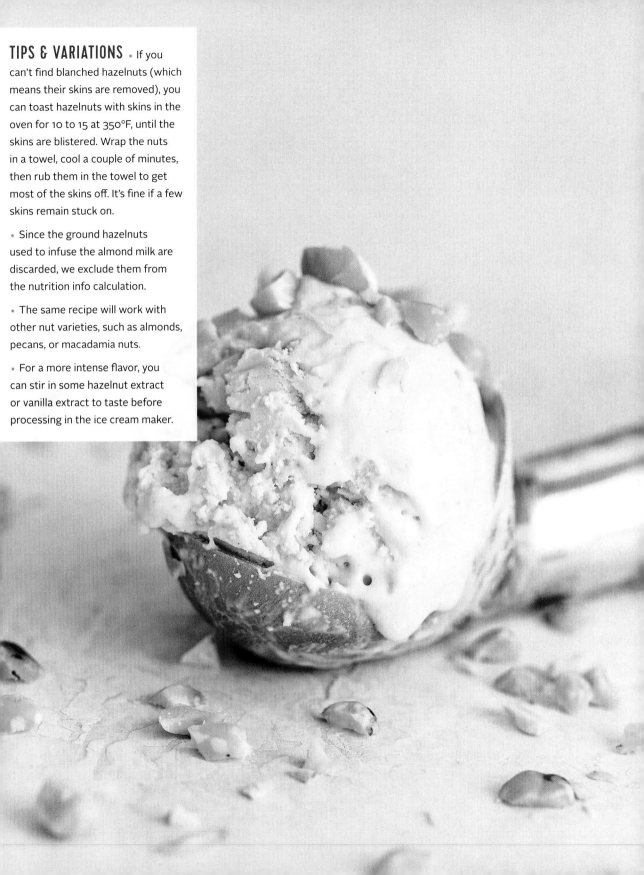

TIPS & VARIATIONS • If you can't find blanched hazelnuts (which means their skins are removed), you can toast hazelnuts with skins in the oven for 10 to 15 at 350°F, until the skins are blistered. Wrap the nuts in a towel, cool a couple of minutes, then rub them in the towel to get most of the skins off. It's fine if a few skins remain stuck on.

• Since the ground hazelnuts used to infuse the almond milk are discarded, we exclude them from the nutrition info calculation.

• The same recipe will work with other nut varieties, such as almonds, pecans, or macadamia nuts.

• For a more intense flavor, you can stir in some hazelnut extract or vanilla extract to taste before processing in the ice cream maker.

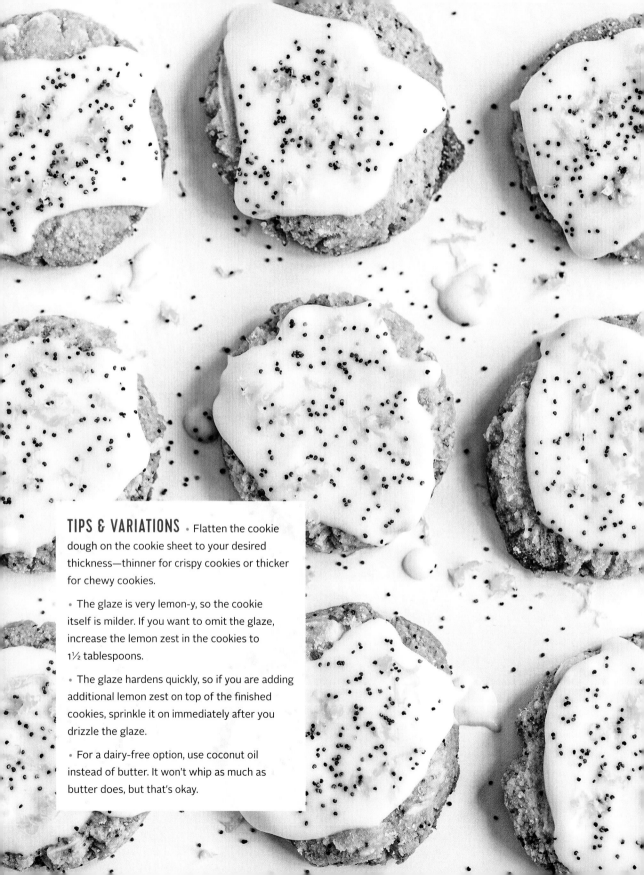

TIPS & VARIATIONS • Flatten the cookie dough on the cookie sheet to your desired thickness—thinner for crispy cookies or thicker for chewy cookies.

• The glaze is very lemon-y, so the cookie itself is milder. If you want to omit the glaze, increase the lemon zest in the cookies to 1½ tablespoons.

• The glaze hardens quickly, so if you are adding additional lemon zest on top of the finished cookies, sprinkle it on immediately after you drizzle the glaze.

• For a dairy-free option, use coconut oil instead of butter. It won't whip as much as butter does, but that's okay.

LEMON POPPY SEED COOKIES

Anything lemon poppy seed reminds me of my favorite coffeehouse. These cookies pair perfectly with an afternoon cup of tea or coffee, and you can easily customize the method to yield either crispy or chewy cookies.

1. Preheat the oven to 350°F. Line a cookie sheet with parchment paper.

2. **Make the cookies:** In a bowl, with an electric hand mixer, beat the butter and erythritol together at medium speed for about 2 minutes, until fluffy. Beat in the gelatin (if using) and vanilla.

3. Beat in the almond flour, ½ cup at a time.

4. Mix in lemon zest and poppy seeds with a spoon or spatula, pressing with the back of the spoon or spatula to incorporate. You can also use your hands to bring it together.

5. Use a medium cookie scoop (~1½ tablespoons) to scoop the dough onto the lined cookie sheet, at least 1½ inches apart. Flatten using your palm.

6. Bake for 13 to 18 minutes, until golden on top. The cookies will still be very soft to the touch. Set aside to cool without moving from the pan.

7. **Meanwhile, make the glaze:** In a small bowl, whisk together the powdered erythritol and lemon juice. If it's too thick for drizzling, thin out with a bit more lemon juice.

8. When the cookies have cooled to warm and are no longer hot, drizzle the glaze over them. Immediately garnish with more lemon zest on top (if using) and poppy seeds. Cool completely to crisp up and set the glaze.

COOKIES

- ½ cup (1 stick) butter, softened at room temperature
- ⅓ cup erythritol
- 1 tablespoon unflavored gelatin powder (optional, but recommended for chewy cookies)
- ½ teaspoon vanilla extract
- 2 cups (8 ounces) blanched almond flour
- 1 tablespoon lemon zest, plus more for garnish (optional)
- 2 teaspoons poppy seeds

GLAZE

- ¼ cup powdered erythritol
- 1 tablespoon lemon juice

MAKES 14 COOKIES

SERVING SIZE
1 cookie (1 ounce)

PER SERVING
154 calories
14 g fat
10 g total carbs
2 g net carbs
4 g protein

CARROT CAKE MUFFINS

Carrots are sometimes excluded from keto recipes due to their higher carb content, but there's no reason not to enjoy them in small amounts if they fit into your macro goals. Here, 1 cup goes a long way, so it doesn't amount to much when divided among 10 muffins. And if you're a fan of carrot cake like I am, these muffins are well worth squeezing into your carbs for the day!

1. Preheat the oven to 350°F. Line 10 cups of a muffin tin with parchment paper liners.

2. In a large bowl, with an electric hand mixer, beat the butter and erythritol at medium speed, until fluffy and light yellow in color.

3. Beat in the cinnamon and vanilla. Beat in the eggs, one at a time.

4. Beat in the almond flour, baking powder, and sea salt until well mixed. (The batter will be very thick, which is normal.)

5. Stir in the grated carrots and 1 cup of the chopped pecans.

6. Divide the batter among the lined muffin cups, filling almost to the top. Sprinkle remaining ½ cup chopped pecans over the muffins. Press gently into the top so that they won't fall off.

7. Bake for 25 to 35 minutes, until the top is golden brown and an inserted toothpick comes out clean. If the top browns before the inside is done, tent with foil and continue to bake until done inside.

8. Cool to firm up the texture before enjoying.

4 *tablespoons (½ stick)* butter

½ *cup* erythritol

2 *teaspoons* ground cinnamon

1 *teaspoon* vanilla extract

3 *large* eggs

3 *cups (12 ounces)* blanched almond flour

2 *teaspoons* baking powder

¼ *teaspoon* sea salt

1 *loosely packed cup (3.5 ounces)* grated carrots

1½ *cups* chopped pecans, divided into 1 cup and ½ cup

MAKES 10 MUFFINS

SERVING SIZE
1 muffin (~3 ounces)

PER SERVING
368 calories
33 g fat
14 g total carbs
6 g net carbs
10 g protein

TIPS & VARIATIONS · If you aren't dairy-free, these are wonderful with cream cheese frosting or glaze. To make it, simply beat together 4 ounces cream cheese, 2 tablespoons butter, ½ cup powdered erythritol, and 1 teaspoon vanilla extract. Then thin out with 1 to 2 tablespoons heavy cream.

· These are buttery, moist muffins. If you cut one open and discover it's not as done as you'd like, you can continue baking the rest of the batch. Just tent the top of the muffin tin with foil and return to the oven in 2- to 3-minute increments.

· For a dairy-free option, use coconut oil instead of the butter. It won't whip as much as butter does, but that's okay.

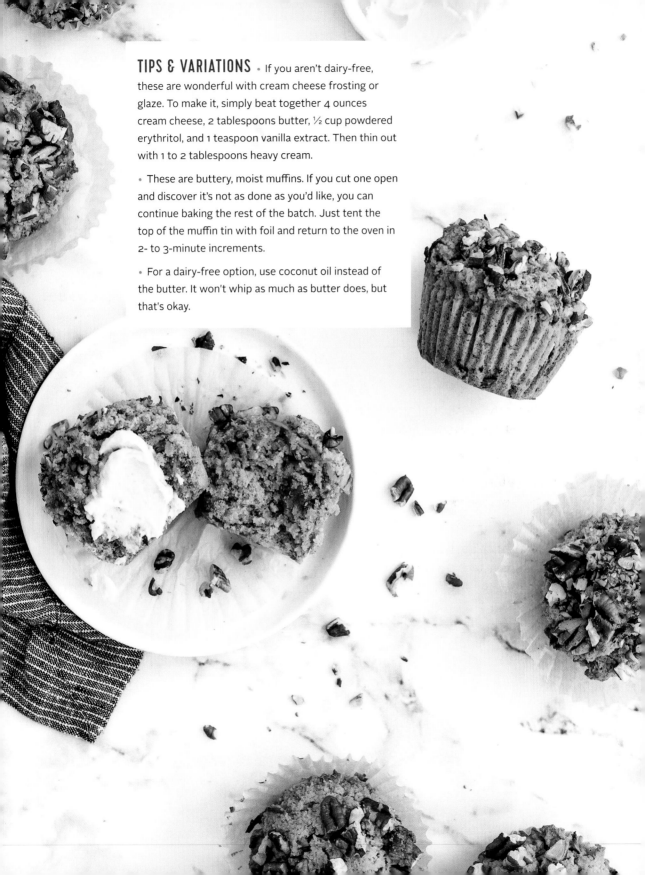

TIPS & VARIATIONS • Like any angel food cake, the most critical part of this recipe is to avoid breaking down the egg whites when folding them into the flour mixture. If they break down, the cake will be too dense.

• If you prefer to make one larger cake instead of using two ramekins, pour all of the batter into one large ovenproof mug or extra-large ramekin (at least 12 ounces). When it is finished baking, you can slice and layer it with whipped cream and strawberries.

• The oven version produces a superior result in both taste and appearance, but the microwave version is much faster.

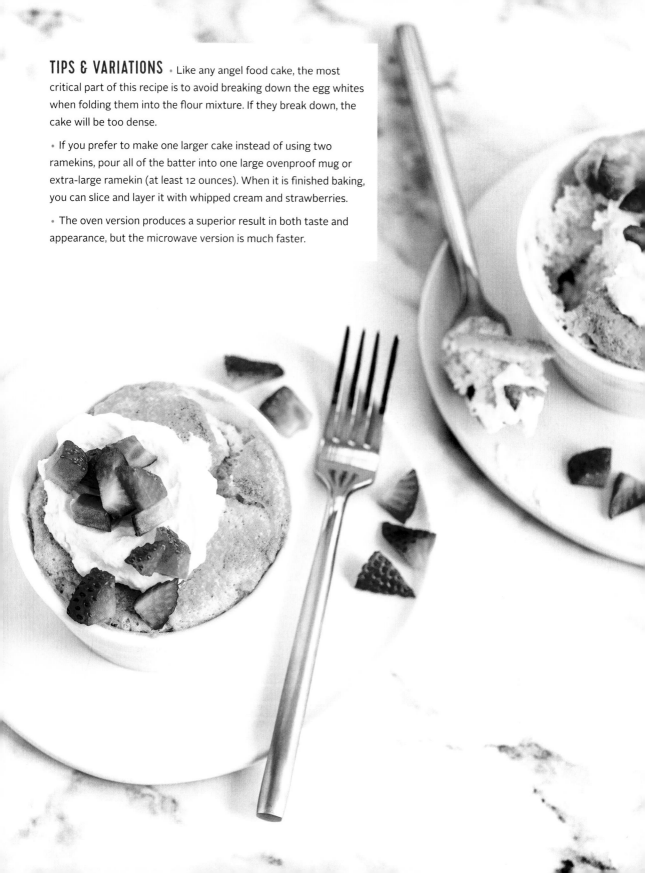

ANGEL FOOD MUG CAKE
WITH STRAWBERRIES

Angel food cake is usually a lighter dessert to begin with, but unfortunately, it's still packed with sugar and flour. This version uses the same method as a traditional angel food cake, but we use keto-friendly ingredients. I also made it even easier for you by turning it into a 2-minute microwave mug cake *or* a 15-minute one in the oven—your choice!

1. If using the oven method, preheat the oven to 350°F.

2. In a medium bowl, with an electric hand mixer, beat the egg whites with the cream of tartar for a couple of minutes at high speed, until stiff peaks form. Beat in the vanilla and almond extract.

3. In another medium bowl, stir together the almond flour, erythritol, and sea salt. Gently fold the flour mixture into the egg whites, being careful not to break them down.

4. Divide the batter between two 4-ounce ramekins or two small mugs.

5. **Oven method:** Place the ramekins in the oven and bake for about 15 minutes, until the tops of the cakes are firm and an inserted toothpick comes out mostly clean (a few crumbs are fine).
   Microwave method: Place the ramekins in the microwave for 70 to 90 seconds, until the tops of the cakes are firm and an inserted toothpick comes out mostly clean (a few crumbs are fine).

6. If desired, garnish with whipped cream (or whipped coconut cream for a dairy-free version). Serve with the sliced strawberries on top.

¼ cup egg whites

Pinch of cream of tartar

¼ teaspoon vanilla extract

$\frac{1}{16}$ teaspoon almond extract (optional)

¼ cup (1 ounce) blanched almond flour

2 tablespoons erythritol

⅛ teaspoon sea salt

Whipped cream or whipped coconut cream, for serving (optional)

¼ cup (1.5 ounces) strawberries, sliced

MAKES 2 SERVINGS

SERVING SIZE

1 cake with strawberry topping (3 ounces), or ½ the recipe

PER SERVING

104 calories

7 g fat

8 g total carbs

3 g net carbs

6 g protein

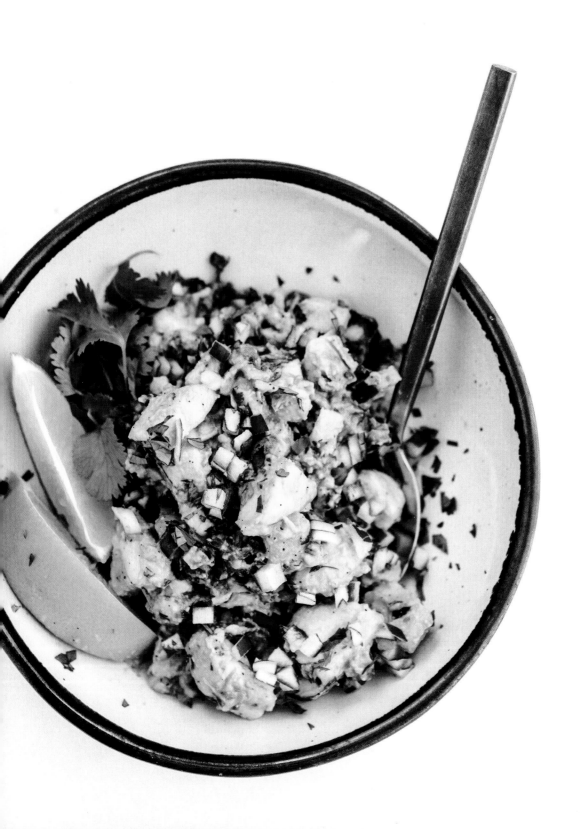

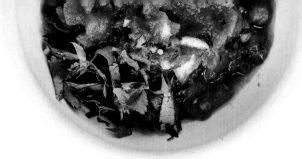

BASIC CONDIMENTS

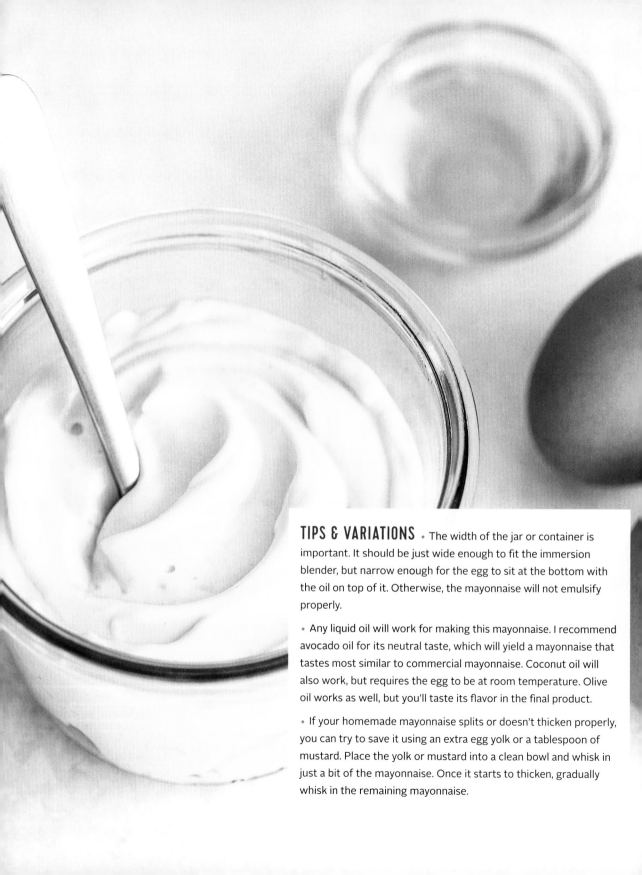

TIPS & VARIATIONS • The width of the jar or container is important. It should be just wide enough to fit the immersion blender, but narrow enough for the egg to sit at the bottom with the oil on top of it. Otherwise, the mayonnaise will not emulsify properly.

• Any liquid oil will work for making this mayonnaise. I recommend avocado oil for its neutral taste, which will yield a mayonnaise that tastes most similar to commercial mayonnaise. Coconut oil will also work, but requires the egg to be at room temperature. Olive oil works as well, but you'll taste its flavor in the final product.

• If your homemade mayonnaise splits or doesn't thicken properly, you can try to save it using an extra egg yolk or a tablespoon of mustard. Place the yolk or mustard into a clean bowl and whisk in just a bit of the mayonnaise. Once it starts to thicken, gradually whisk in the remaining mayonnaise.

2-MINUTE AVOCADO OIL MAYONNAISE

So many brands of store-bought mayonnaise are filled with questionable ingredients. Sugar? Soy? Starch? No thanks! There's no reason to put up with all of those ingredients when you can easily make your own homemade mayonnaise in under 5 minutes. All you need are these 5 ingredients, a jar, and an immersion blender!

1. Crack the egg into the bottom of a tall glass jar. (You can also use a tall drinking glass, but make sure it's wide enough for an immersion blender to fit. Do not use a bowl.)

2. Add the mustard, vinegar, and sea salt on top of the egg, trying not to disturb the egg. Do not whisk or stir.

3. Pour the oil on top. Again, do not whisk or stir.

4. Carefully submerge an immersion blender into the bottom of the jar so that it's right where the egg is. Blend on low power for about 20 seconds without moving, until you see most of the jar has turned white. Then slowly start to move the blender upward, without lifting the blender out into the air. Once you reach the top of the oil, slowly move back down to the bottom. Go up and down like this a few times, until mayonnaise forms.

5. Store the mayonnaise right in the jar, in the refrigerator, for 7 to 10 days.

1 *large* egg

1 *teaspoon* Dijon mustard

2 *teaspoons* apple cider vinegar

¼ *teaspoon* sea salt

1 *cup* avocado oil

MAKES 1¼ CUPS

SERVING SIZE
1 tablespoon (~0.6 ounce)

PER SERVING
100 calories
11 g fat
0 g total carbs
0 g net carbs
0 g protein

BASIC CONDIMENTS

RANCH DRESSING

If there's one keto dressing recipe to master, this is it! Every single person I've shared this with has sworn it's better than the most popular household favorite ranch from the store—without any sugar, refined oils, preservatives, or processed ingredients. It takes just a few minutes to whip up, stores well in the fridge for 7 to 10 days, and is great for everything from salads to dipping to casseroles!

1. In a medium bowl, whisk all the ingredients together, except the almond milk.

2. Add the almond milk gradually, until you reach the desired consistency (use less if you want this to be a thick dip, more if you want a thinner dressing).

3. Refrigerate for at least 1 hour to let the flavors develop.

TIPS & VARIATIONS · You can use ranch dressing as a dip or as salad dressing—this recipe makes a consistency that works for both. You may need less almond milk for an extra-thick dip, or more for a thinner dressing.

· Ranch dressing may thicken more if it sits in the fridge for a long time. You can thin it out with more almond milk when needed.

· For a nut-free version, you can replace unsweetened almond milk with coconut milk or heavy cream.

· This recipe uses dried herbs for convenience, but you can also use fresh if you'd like. You'll need 1 tablespoon fresh herbs to replace each teaspoon dried herbs.

1 *cup* 2-Minute Avocado Oil Mayonnaise (page 235)

½ *cup* sour cream

2 *teaspoons* lemon juice

2 *teaspoons* dried parsley

1 *teaspoon* dried dill

1 *teaspoon* dried chives

½ *teaspoon* garlic powder

½ *teaspoon* onion powder

½ *teaspoon* sea salt

¼ *teaspoon* black pepper

¼ *cup* unsweetened almond milk

MAKES 1½ CUPS

SERVING SIZE
2 tablespoons (~1 ounce)

PER SERVING
155 calories
16 g fat
0 g total carbs
0 g net carbs
0 g protein

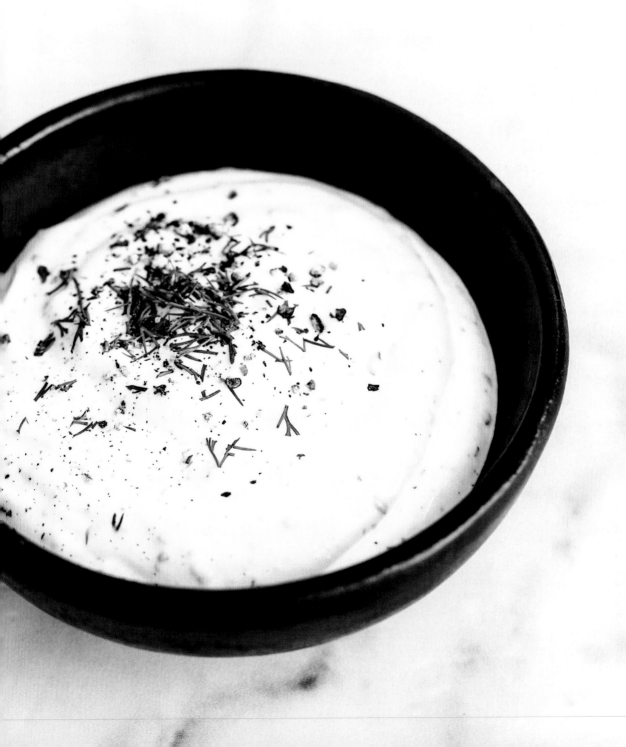

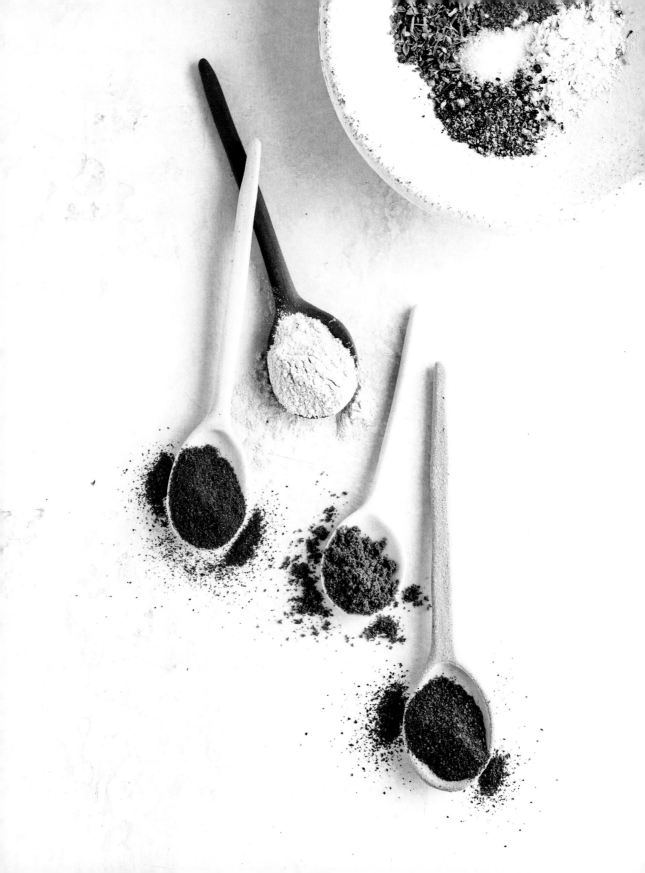

TACO SEASONING

Did you know that many store-bought seasoning mixes contain added sugar and starch? You can find ones that don't, but you don't have to, because making your own is *so easy*! I always keep a small glass jar of this stuff around. And you can see how much I love it, because it's an ingredient in multiple recipes in this book!

1. In a small bowl or jar, stir all the ingredients together.

2. Store the taco seasoning in an airtight container in the pantry.

> **TIPS & VARIATIONS** • If you don't have smoked paprika or dried oregano, you can substitute these with regular paprika or dried cilantro, respectively.
>
> • This makes a moderately mild taco seasoning. If you like it spicy, increase the cayenne pepper to ¼ teaspoon.
>
> • To use the taco seasoning for taco meat, brown the ground beef first. Then add 2 tablespoons seasoning and ½ cup water per pound of meat. Simmer until the extra liquid evaporates or absorbs into the meat.
>
> • Serving size is based on the amount of taco seasoning used for a serving of meat, ¼ pound. The recipe makes enough seasoning for 3 pounds of meat.

2 *tablespoons* chili powder

1 *tablespoon* ground cumin

1 *tablespoon* sea salt

½ *tablespoon* black pepper

½ *tablespoon* smoked paprika

1 *teaspoon* dried oregano

1 *teaspoon* garlic powder

½ *teaspoon* onion powder

⅛ *teaspoon* cayenne pepper

MAKES 6 TABLESPOONS

SERVING SIZE
½ tablespoon (0.1 ounce)

PER SERVING
8 calories
0 g fat
1 g total carbs
1 g net carbs
0 g protein

PANTRY STAPLE SALSA

Restaurant-style salsa is actually super simple to make at home! Most of the ingredients for this recipe are pantry staples, making it easy to make at the last minute. It's delicious for dipping, and also a fabulous ingredient in a variety of recipes, like Slow Cooker Creamy Salsa Chicken (page 126) or Chicken Quesadillas (page 62).

1. In a food processor, combine all the ingredients.

2. Pulse, scraping down the sides with a spatula, until desired consistency is reached.

3. Adjust the salt and chili powder (if using) to taste, pulsing 1 to 2 times again to combine.

TIPS & VARIATIONS • Omit the chili powder for mild salsa, or add to taste for spicier salsa. Keep in mind that green chilies in the canned tomatoes already add some heat to this recipe. If you are unsure, start by making the salsa without chili powder first, then taste to see if you want more heat.

• Be careful not to overprocess. You want to have some chunks left in the tomatoes.

• You can use red or white onion to your liking. Red onions are slightly higher in carbs.

3¾ cups (30 ounces) canned no-salt-added diced tomatoes with green chilies, drained

¼ cup (1.5 ounces) chopped onion

¼ cup chopped fresh cilantro

2 cloves garlic, coarsely chopped

1½ tablespoons lime juice

½ teaspoon sea salt, or to taste

⅛ teaspoon chili powder (optional; see Tips & Variations)

MAKES 2½ CUPS

SERVING SIZE
¼ cup (2.5 ounces)

PER SERVING
19 calories
0 g fat
4 g total carbs
4 g net carbs
0 g protein

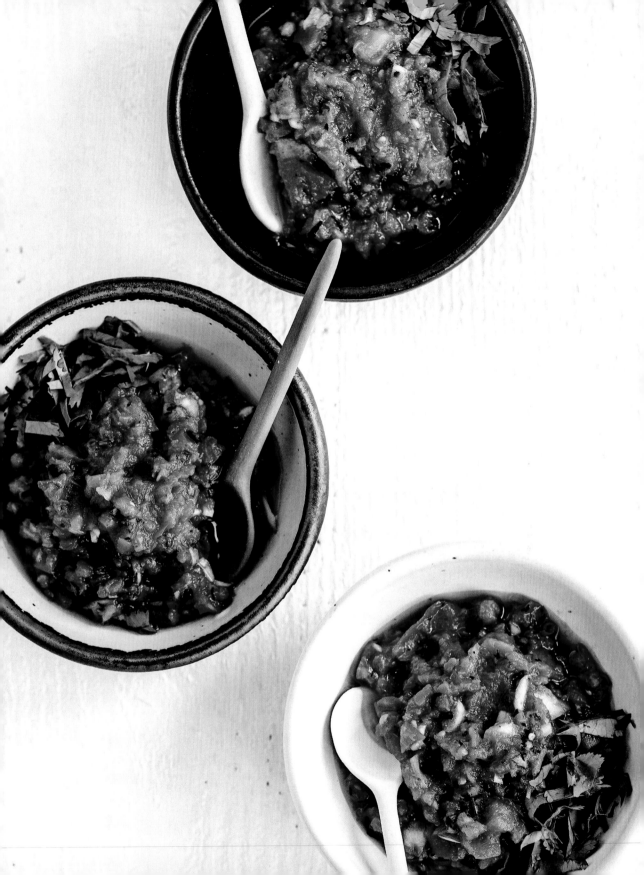

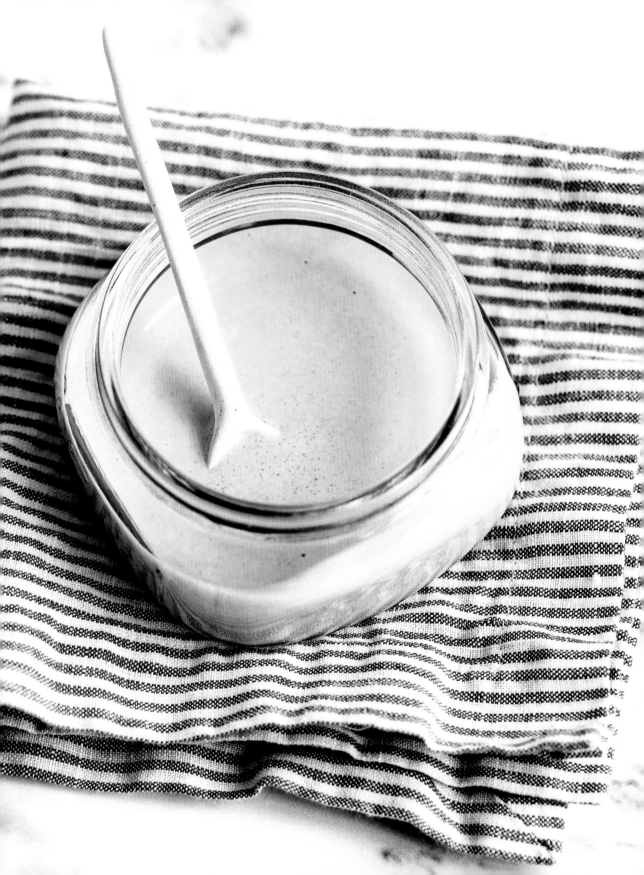

SUGAR-FREE "HONEY" MUSTARD

Of course, real honey mustard is made with honey, which isn't suitable for a keto lifestyle. But you might be surprised that many honey-mustard dressings and dips don't actually have any honey in them anyway. It turns out that you can easily re-create that classic honey-mustard flavor using sugar-free sweetener and other natural ingredients. The best part? You can do it in under 5 minutes!

¾ *cup* 2-Minute Avocado Oil Mayonnaise (page 235)

⅓ *cup* Dijon mustard (or regular yellow mustard)

⅓ *cup* powdered erythritol

1 *tablespoon* apple cider vinegar

Pinch of sea salt

Pinch of cayenne pepper

MAKES 1¼ CUPS

In a medium bowl, whisk together all the ingredients until smooth.

TIPS & VARIATIONS • If you're using this sauce as a salad dressing, you can thin it out by whisking in 2 teaspoons olive oil and 1 additional teaspoon apple cider vinegar for each ½ cup of sugar-free "honey" mustard.

• If you'll be storing the honey mustard, you can use fewer dishes by simply putting all the ingredients in a small jar and shaking to combine. Cover the jar and refrigerate.

SERVING SIZE
2 tablespoons (1 ounce)

PER SERVING
125 calories
13 g fat
5 g total carbs
0 g net carbs
0 g protein

BASIC CONDIMENTS

RASPBERRY SAUCE

I first made sugar-free raspberry sauce to use as a topping for Classic Cheesecake (page 210), but it's just as delicious over a multitude of other desserts. With only 3 ingredients and a quick cooking time, this recipe will be ready in only about 10 minutes!

12 ounces (2⅔ cups) raspberries

2 tablespoons lemon juice

⅓ cup powdered erythritol, or to taste

MAKES 1 CUP

SERVING SIZE
2 tablespoons (~1.3 ounces)

PER SERVING
22 calories
0 g fat
11 g total carbs
3 g net carbs
0 g protein

1. In a small saucepan, combine the raspberries, lemon juice, and powdered erythritol. Cook over medium-low heat for 2 to 3 minutes, until the raspberries start to soften.

2. Adjust the heat to a gentle simmer, mash the berries with the back of a spoon, and continue cooking for 5 to 8 minutes, until thickened. Adjust the sweetener to taste. The sauce will thicken more as it cools.

TIPS & VARIATIONS • You can use any kind of berries you like for this recipe, but raspberries (along with blackberries) are the lowest in carbs. Cooking times may need to be adjusted if using another type of berry.

• The exact volume of sauce you get will depend on how much you reduce it. The longer it cooks, the more moisture evaporates, so it gets thicker and reduces in volume.

• For a flavor twist, try adding ½ teaspoon vanilla extract or 1 tablespoon orange zest.

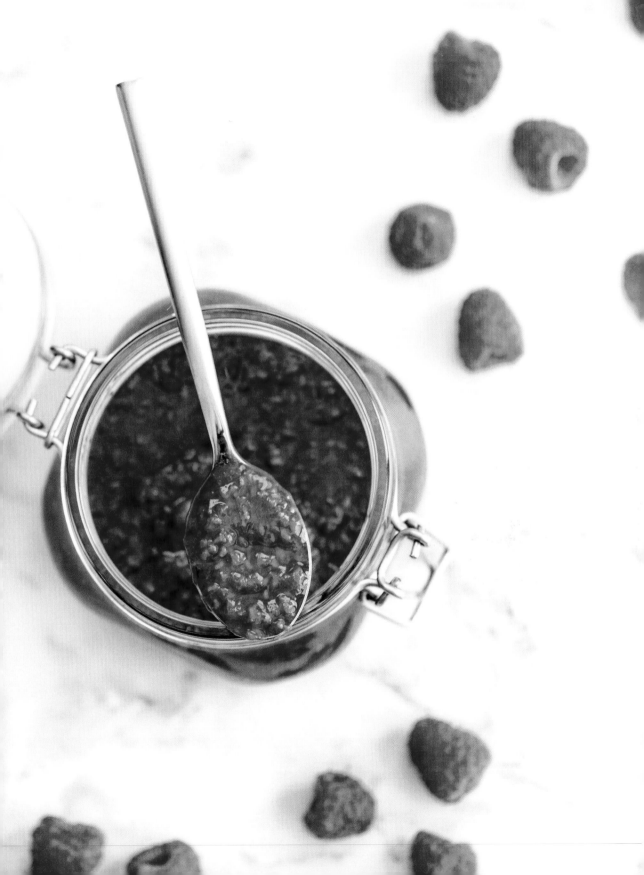

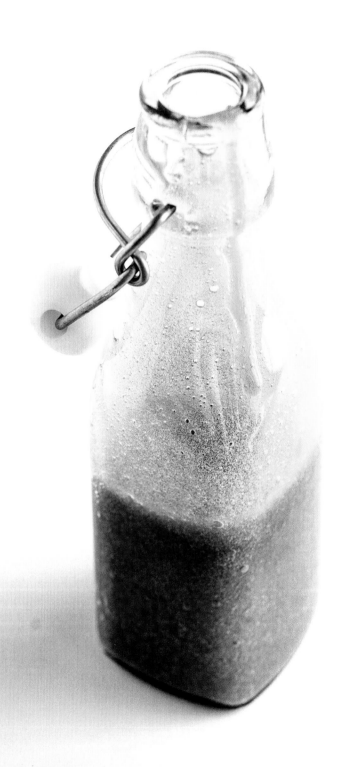

HOMEMADE SUGAR-FREE MAPLE SYRUP

A tall stack of (keto!) pancakes just isn't complete without maple syrup. But as we all know, real maple syrup is basically just sugar. It's simply a no-go for a keto lifestyle. Fortunately, there is a way to make your own keto-friendly maple syrup replacement at home. You can get all the delicious maple flavor—naturally!—by using maple extract and a natural sugar-free sweetener.

1 cup water

1 cup powdered erythritol

1½ tablespoons real maple extract

½ teaspoon xanthan gum

MAKES 1 CUP

SERVING SIZE
2 tablespoons (1.2 ounces)

PER SERVING
0 calories
0 g fat
18 g total carbs
0 g net carbs
0 g protein

1. In a small saucepan, whisk together the water, powdered erythritol, and maple extract. Bring the mixture to a gentle boil and simmer for about 5 minutes, stirring occasionally, until the erythritol mostly dissolves.

2. Pour the liquid into a blender. Sprinkle half of the xanthan gum on top (don't dump, just sprinkle lightly and evenly to avoid clumping). Puree immediately, and continue until no lumps remain. Repeat with the remaining xanthan gum.

3. Wait a few minutes to allow the syrup to thicken further. If it's still thinner than you'd like, add a little more xanthan gum (1/16 teaspoon at a time, using half of a 1/8-teaspoon measuring spoon, sprinkled lightly and pureed again).

TIPS & VARIATIONS • It's highly recommended to use real maple extract, not the imitation kind that has an artificial flavor and aftertaste.

• Xanthan gum clumps easily when it hits liquid, which is why it's so critical to sprinkle and not dump it in. It also takes some time to thicken and can get slimy if you overdo it, so err on the side of using less and add just a tiny bit more at a time to achieve your desired consistency.

BASIC CONDIMENTS

SIMPLE GUACAMOLE

No Mexican meal is complete without some amazing guac! I became obsessed with adding it to my burrito bowls (without rice or beans, of course) at my favorite Mexican place years ago, and started making my own shortly after. Even for novice cooks, fresh homemade guacamole is super simple to make from scratch.

1. Scoop the avocados into a medium bowl. Add jalapeño, onion, cilantro, lime juice, garlic, sea salt, and black pepper, and mash together using a fork or potato masher.

2. Adjust the sea salt, black pepper, lime juice, and jalapeño to taste.

TIPS & VARIATIONS • Feel free to customize the amount of lime juice, jalapeño, sea salt, and black pepper you use to suit your palate—guacamole is super simple to adjust to taste.

• The jalapeño seeds and ribs have the most heat, so omit them for milder guacamole that still has some jalapeño flavor.

2 *medium* avocados (6 ounces each)

¼ *medium* jalapeño pepper, finely diced

¼ *cup (1.3 ounces)* finely diced red onion

3 *packed tablespoons* fresh cilantro, chopped

2 *tablespoons* lime juice

1 *clove* garlic, minced

½ *teaspoon* sea salt

¼ *teaspoon* black pepper

MAKES 2 CUPS

SERVING SIZE
¼ cup (3 ounces)

PER SERVING
84 calories
7 g fat
5 g total carbs
2 g net carbs
1 g protein

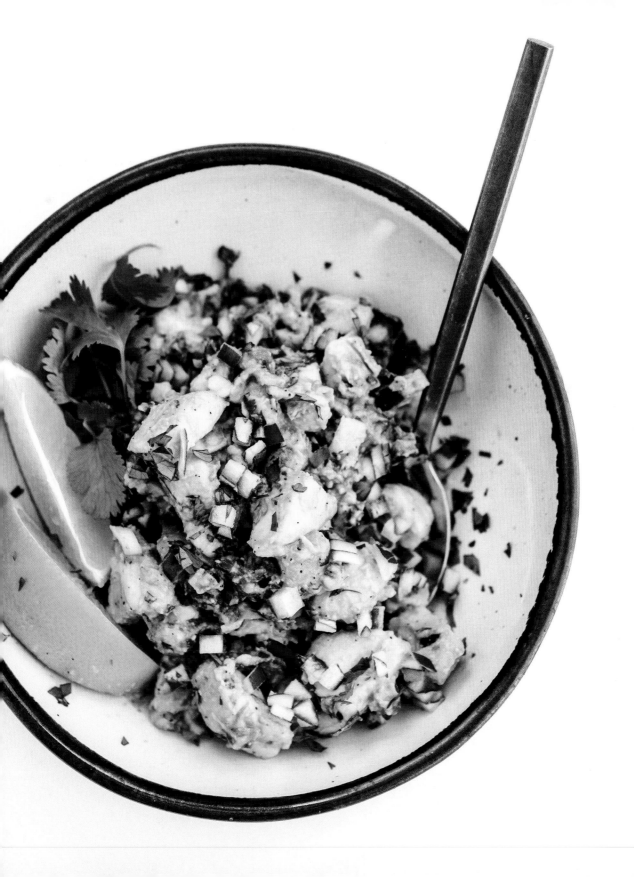

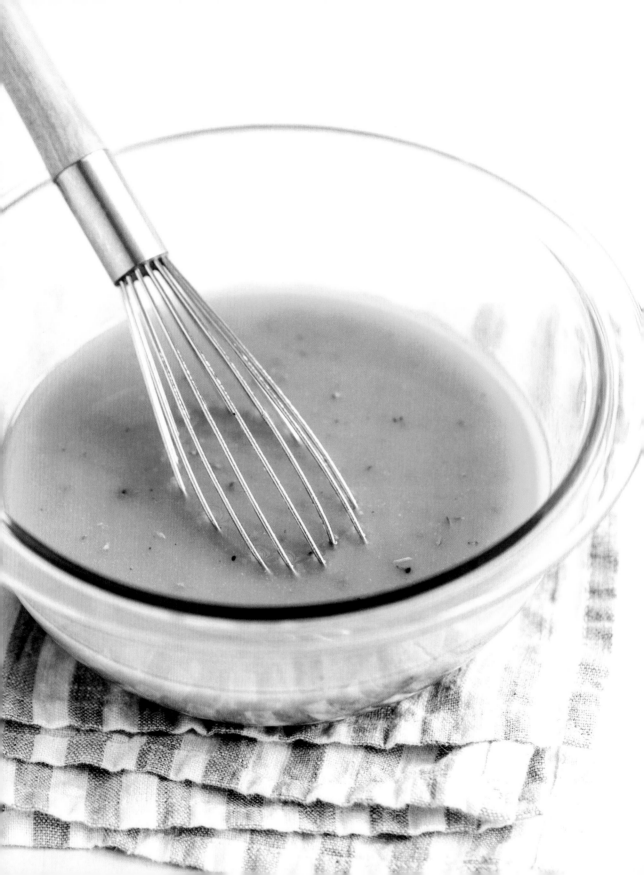

BASIC GREEK VINAIGRETTE

When you want to keep your salad dressing light, dairy-free, and still packed with healthy fats for a keto lifestyle, a basic Greek vinaigrette is a perfect choice. It pairs perfectly with Greek salad, but is also versatile enough for many other types of salads, including Greek Horiatiki Zucchini Salad (page 94). And you can usually store it for a couple of weeks!

In a small bowl, whisk together all the ingredients until smooth.

TIPS & VARIATIONS • I recommend 1 tablespoon dressing to every 1 to 1½ cups salad. If your salad has greens, a serving of salad will be 2 to 3 cups, so about 2 tablespoons dressing will go with it. For a salad without greens, a serving will be smaller (typically about 1 cup), so 1 tablespoon dressing should be sufficient for a serving.

• Like any vinaigrette, this dressing may separate after storing in the fridge for a while. Simply shake it to re-emulsify.

⅓ *cup* olive oil

1 *tablespoon* red wine vinegar

1 *tablespoon* lemon juice

1 *teaspoon* Dijon mustard

½ *teaspoon* dried oregano

¼ *teaspoon* garlic powder

¼ *teaspoon* sea salt

⅛ *teaspoon* black pepper

MAKES ~½ CUP

SERVING SIZE
2 tablespoons (~¾ ounce)

PER SERVING
162 calories
18 g fat
0 g total carbs
0 g net carbs
0 g protein

BIBLIOGRAPHY

Hu, T., Bazzano, L.A. "The Low-Carbohydrate Diet and Cardiovascular Risk Factors: Evidence from Epidemiologic Studies." *Nutrition, Metabolism and Cardiovascular Diseases*, Volume 24, Issue 4 (2014): 337–343, www.ncbi .nlm.nih.gov/pmc/articles/PMC4351995.

Hu, T., et al. "The Effects of a Low-Carbohydrate Diet on Appetite: A Randomized Controlled Trial." *Nutrition, Metabolism, and Cardiovascular Diseases*: NMCD, U.S. National Library of Medicine, June 2016, www.ncbi.nlm .nih.gov/pubmed/26803589.

Paoli, A., Rubini, A., Volek, J.S., Grimaldi, K.A. "Beyond Weight Loss: A Review of the Therapeutic Uses of Very-Low-Carbohydrate (Ketogenic) Diets." *European Journal of Clinical Nutrition*, 2014, www.ncbi.nlm.nih.gov/pmc/ articles/PMC3826507.

Roberts, M.N., Megan, N., et al. "A Ketogenic Diet Extends Longevity and Healthspan in Adult Mice." *Cell Metabolism*, U.S. National Library of Medicine, Sept. 5, 2017, www.ncbi.nlm.nih.gov/ pubmed/28877457.

THANK YOU

Writing a book has been a dream of mine since I was a little girl, and many years later, writing it has filled my heart with immense gratitude. I couldn't have done it without the amazing people in my life who made this possible.

To my readers: You are the reason I do what I do every day, and the reason this book exists. Your struggles and success stories touch my soul, your feedback pushes me to make the best for you, and I am elated every single time one of you makes my recipes. It brings me so much joy to hear that my creations help you—it's my greatest measurement of success. Thank you from the bottom of my heart for supporting me, for listening to me, and for letting me be a part of your life.

To my husband, Oleg: You are the love of my life, my best friend, my business partner, my biggest supporter, my toughest critic, and my rock—all at the same time. Thank you for supporting my dreams. I am so grateful that you brought me out of a dark time in my life, and beyond excited that you recently took the leap of faith to leave your job so that we can work on building our castles in the air together. You are now truly my partner in every way possible. I absolutely *cannot wait* to see all the other amazing things we will create. Thank you for being you and getting me like no one else does.

To my two little girls, Bella and Gaby:
Thank you for your unparalleled enthusiasm stirring every bowl in the kitchen and for being my most critical taste testers.

To my mom and dad: Thank you for raising me to be fearless and determined, even in ways you didn't expect, and for sticking by me even when it was tough. I see both of you in myself every day. I know it wasn't easy for an immigrant family of engineers to understand how a software engineer turned into an entrepreneur, writer, photographer, recipe developer, business strategist, marketer, project manager, and wearer of many other hats behind the scenes. Earning your respect and understanding of what I do has been the most rewarding experience, and your support and encouragement mean the world to me.

To my culinary assistant, Emily Dingmann:
Thank you for the long days in the kitchen and for being my sounding board for the crazy ideas Oleg and I have, food related and otherwise. You do things better than I hope for, you understand my blogging journey, and working with you brings me so much joy. Thanks for your enthusiasm, dedication, and useful tips, and for reminding me that the odd things our same-age kids do are totally normal. And I appreciate your help in making the Wholesome Yum Meal Plans a reality.

To my amazing agent, Stacey Glick: Thank you for believing in me and pushing me to submit my book proposal. I so appreciate you taking the time to answer all my tough questions, read my lengthy emails, ease my concerns, give me the honest truth, and be my relentless advocate. You have made my dream of being a published author a reality.

To my talented food photographer and food stylist, Ashley McLaughlin, and her awesome team, Leanne Ray and Wes Park: Thank you for working tirelessly to bring my recipes to life in the most beautiful way ever. I appreciate your flexibility on our crazy, tight timeline, your accommodation of my detailed requests, and the opportunity to learn from you at the photo shoot.

To the Wholesome Yum Team, past and present: Elena, Amanda, Noelle, Kelley, Lesley, Felicia, Chantal, Pie, Tiffany, Holly, Jovita, Yumna, Tammy, Michelle, Ivy, Clare, Lara, Dino, Stacey, Monica, Julie, Wendy, Jen, Nita, Lisa, and Laura—thank you for your help with the various moving pieces at Wholesome Yum! To my recipe tester, Helen Baldus, I appreciate your meticulous testing and detailed, actionable feedback.

To my product business partner, Jeffrey Lager: Thank you for believing in what we can do together. I am beyond excited!

To the Penguin Random House team:
Thank you for taking a chance on me and publishing my work. To my brilliant literary editors, Dervla Kelly and Alyse Diamond, I am so grateful for your support of my vision for this book, and for helping me make it everything I dreamed of and more. To Katherine, Brianne, Stephanie, Francesca, Christina, Danielle, Lindsey, Tammy, Heather, Kim, Joyce, Zoe, and the entire Penguin Random House editorial, marketing, design, and publicity teams, thank you for your hard work in making my book beautiful and helping me share it with the world.

INDEX

Copyright © 2019 by Maya Krampf

All rights reserved.
Published in the United States by Harmony Books, an imprint of Random House, a division of Penguin Random House LLC, New York.
harmonybooks.com

Harmony Books is a registered trademark, and the Circle colophon is a trademark of Penguin Random House LLC.

Library of Congress Cataloging-in-Publication Data is available upon request.

ISBN 978-1-9848-2662-6
Ebook ISBN 978-1-9848-2663-3

Printed in the United States of America

Book and cover design by Jennifer K. Beal Davis
Photographs by Ashley McLaughlin
Author photograph by Oleg Krampf

10 9 8 7 6 5 4 3 2

First Edition